Breaking the Silence on
Women's Hair Loss

D0557024

Breaking the Silence on
Women's Hair Loss

Candace Hoffmann

Copyright © 2006 Candace Hoffmann

All rights reserved. No part of this publication may be reproduced, stored in a retrieval system, or transmitted in any form without the prior permission of the copyright owner.

For ordering information and bulk order discounts, contact:
Woodland Publishing
448 East 800 North, Orem, UT 84097
Toll-free telephone: (800) 777-BOOK (2665)

Please visit our Web site: www.woodlandpublishing.com

Note: The information in this book is for educational purposes only and is not recommended as a means of diagnosing or treating an illness. All matters concerning physical and mental health should be supervised by a health practitioner knowledgeable in treating that particular condition. Neither the publisher nor the author directly or indirectly dispenses medical advice, nor do they prescribe any remedies or assume any responsibility for those who choose to treat themselves.

A cataloging-in-publication record for this book is available from the Library of Congress.

ISBN 10: 1-58054-467-3
ISBN 13: 978-1-58054-467-2

Printed in the United States of America

06 07 08 09 10 1 2 3 4 5 6 7 8 9 20

To my father,
Harold (Chic) Henion
(1911–2004)

Contents

Acknowledgments

Books do not write themselves, and this one is no exception. I am less the author of this book and more a facilitator, helping to give a voice to one of the last taboos: women's hair loss. To that end, I thank:

The nearly one hundred women from around the world who shared their stories with me. You are, and you remain, my inspiration.

Kevin and Laura, founders of HairLossTalk.com and HerAlopecia.com, respectively, for their invaluable help.

Anita Bhorjee, for her careful review of the manuscript and her invaluable suggestions, and for allowing me to use parts of her manuscript "10 Hair Loss Myths."

The medical experts who took the time to talk with me and walk me through some of the more difficult aspects of treatment and diagnosis.

My husband, Michael, who always thinks I can do whatever I set out to do, however crazy, and who loves me, often in spite of myself.

My children, Gregory and Gabrielle, who never fail to keep me grounded. I love you both dearly.

My mother, who kept asking, "How is the book coming?" and encouraged me through what was, for both of us, our darkest year.

James Gaffney, my best friend, who, knowing the lonely journey of writing a book, never ceases to lend me his courage when I have none left of my own.

Introduction

"No one dies from hair loss, do they? Two years ago, over a course of about eight months, I lost all my hair," a seventeen-year-old wrote to me. "I was put on antidepressants and tried to commit suicide three times. I hated the way I looked. I hated the way others felt bad for me."

Every day in America, thirty million women—one out of every four—are coping with hair loss, and, for the most part, they are suffering like this young woman, alone and in silence.

Consider these figures from the American Academy of Dermatology (AAD): For every five men with hereditary hair loss, there are three women who are also losing their hair. But women's hair loss, the organization says, "remains a 'taboo' subject for the media, the public and patients," and worse, the medical profession often does not take it seriously.

As a medical journalist, and as a woman coping with genetic hair loss, I felt I was more than capable of sifting through the tangle of information and misinformation available on women's hair loss. And while I didn't for a minute think this would be easy, I was not prepared for the enormous undertaking that lay before me.

I realized I had not really grasped the reality of women's hair loss once I began receiving responses to a survey I sent out via two Web sites—www. HairLossTalk.com and its sister Web site, www. HerAlopecia.com. I received e-mail responses, my fax machine spat out pages, and handwritten replies turned up in my mailbox. Nearly one hundred women of all ages from all over the United States, Canada, Europe, and Asia responded with stories of frustration and suffering.

"I lose a little bit of sanity every morning in the shower," a twenty-seven-year-old woman writes.

"It has been a personal struggle. At first, denial. How could a seventeen-year-old be losing her hair, especially from genetic factors? I thought only old men had this problem," a twenty-year-old says of her now three-year ordeal.

"I am beyond thin hair; you see my scalp," says a thirty-seven-year-old.

One fifty-three-year-old woman who survived a near-fatal car crash that left her comatose for three days says, "I came through that quite broken-up and scarred, but yet never felt as disfigured and ugly, even with a three-inch scar on my forehead, as I have since my hair loss."

"I've fought hair loss really hard, but I'm losing," writes another, a forty-one-year-old who is considering buying a wig. She notes that she's read every hair loss book available and not one offers any hope.

This response, of course, gave me pause.

What do I have to offer her with this book? There are some forms of women's hair loss for which there are no "cures," even though some articles and books that are available would make it seem there are. And then I realized what I could offer.

A voice.

If a fatal illness were affecting thirty million women, it would grab the attention of science and the public. There would be marathon races, fund-raisers, searches for a cure, and ribbons to wear on lapels. It would have a voice.

"I almost wish it were caused by chemotherapy [treatment for cancer]," a twenty-seven-year-old woman says. "I know that sounds horrible to say, but hair loss caused by chemo is explainable and accepted by society."

No, nobody dies from hair loss, but it is life-altering.

The women who took the time to write poured their hearts out telling me their experiences. Some told me they no longer hold jobs; others are so depressed they feel there is no hope; some feel they will never marry or, if married, will lose their husbands. Many women say they are not just betrayed by the medical profession; they are not even being heard. They feel abandoned and ignored.

One woman, age fifty-seven, queried her doctor about hair loss, and he placated her by saying that in all his years of practice he'd never seen a bald-headed woman. "He didn't realize I was wearing a wig," she told me.

Many of these women have spent thousands of dollars going to doctor after doctor, often getting conflicting diagnoses. They spend their money on topical treatments, shampoos, volumizers, vitamins, herbs, and devices that hold the implied promise of hair growth or enhancement.

"I'd put dog poop on my head if I thought it would grow hair," one young woman says. I was surprised at the number of women in their twenties and thirties who wrote to me. But I shouldn't have been.

The AAD estimates that of those thirty million American women suffering with hair loss, ten million, or one-third, are under age forty.

Ironically, this may be a good thing. Unlike their mothers and grandmothers, young women are not quite so likely to keep silent about this. After all, we can offer them the prospect of growing old without wrinkles, droopy eyelids, or sagging jaw lines; is it any surprise they are now asking that in growing old they keep their hair too?

One has to ask this question: Is women's hair loss simply a cosmetic concern, like droopy eyelids? Pfizer, the pharmaceutical company that makes Rogaine (topical minoxidil), the only topical treatment approved by the Food and Drug Administration (FDA) for the treatment of hair loss, found in a survey that women would rather gain fifteen pounds than lose their hair.

A physician writing in the *Harvard Men's Health Watch* (November 2002) outlined the various treatment options for men in treating their own hair loss, pointed out the pros and cons of using the treatments available, and ended the article this way: "From a medical point of view, there is no need to treat normal hair loss. At best, the treatments are only partially effective, and although they are generally safe, some men may experience side effects. Take a look in the mirror and think it over. And before you decide, try to imagine how Michael Jordan would look with a bit of hair."

Who is our Michael Jordan?

While there may not be a celebrity bald-headed woman as our role model, we do have each other. We are a sisterhood thirty million strong, and it is time we are heard. And that's why I've written this book.

I suspect that if thirty million women actually suffer with discernible hair loss, it's just the tip of the iceberg. Look at it this way: If one out of every four women is truly losing her hair, the other three women are worrying about their own hair.

Isn't it time we began talking about it?

1

Hair in Myth and Legend

Hair—what's a woman without it? Images of beauty are often linked to our locks. Fairy tales, myths, and legends abound with hair central to the story. Think of fair Rapunzel, condemned by a nasty witch to solitary life in a tower until a prince traveling through the forest hears her glorious voice and beckons her to let down her hair—hair so long and strong that he is able to climb it for their secret tryst. Then the witch blocks the hair apparent's ascent by cutting off Rapunzel's hair and thus, for a while—before the happy-ever-after ending—cuts off her identity.

Remember O. Henry's poignant story of Christmas selflessness—"The Gift of the Magi"? A young couple, so in love, want to give each other a special Christmas gift—he, a set of tortoise-shell combs for her beautiful hair; she, a fob for his precious watch. But alas, they are too poor for even such simple gifts. Unbeknownst to each other, they hit upon an idea.

She decides to cut off her flowing hair and sell it in order to buy the watch fob, and he sells his watch in order to have enough money to buy the combs. At the end of the story we do not mourn his loss of the watch so much as her loss of hair.

Then there is the story of Berenice, a queen in ancient Egypt known for her beautiful hair. Her husband, Ptolemy III, went off to war; Berenice asked the gods to watch over him and keep him safe, and then she made a bargain. She would cut off her hair if the gods would return her husband safely to her. She cut her tresses and lay them on the altar of Venus. Sure enough, King Ptolemy returned safe and sound. Some accounts of the story say the king was very angry at finding his wife's hair gone. When he went to the temple to view the hair he loved so much, it had disappeared.

The court astronomers told him that the gods were so impressed with her sacrifice that they placed Berenice's locks in the sky, where they became a swirl of stars, and said that the distraught king could view them whenever he looked at the night sky. Coma Berenices is a constellation of stars located between the constellations Virgo and Ursa Major and can be seen in the northern hemisphere in spring and summer.

For women who are losing their hair, such stories cut to the quick. The sheering of Rapunzel's locks, her identity, was the ultimate indignity, the loss of what little power she had. For the young woman in O. Henry's story, cutting her hair was a sacrifice for love, as was Berenice's, who used it to bargain with the gods.

Wonderful, luxurious hair is seen all around us. For some actresses, their hair is as famous as they are—sometimes more so. Farrah Fawcett's hair in the 1970s held us spellbound; Jennifer Aniston's coiffure launched new styles in the 1990s. Meg Ryan, Heather Locklear, Daryl Hannah, Oprah Winfrey, Halle Barry, Sophia Loren are but a few actresses whose manes are nearly as famous as their work. You can easily walk into a hair salon and say, "Give me a Meg Ryan" or "a Halle Barry," and be understood. Well, some women can; those of us with hair loss can't, at least not without modifications.

Pfizer's survey, which revealed women would rather gain weight than lose their hair, presented a hypothetical choice. The women answering it were likely not actually faced with the reality of hair loss. But those of us who are losing our hair are dealing daily with a harsh reality. We don't have to guess which lesser evil we'd prefer.

Can we bargain with the gods like Berenice? Give us back our hair, and tack on that extra fifteen pounds? Give us back our hair, and we'll promise to be better people? Give us back our hair, and we'll tithe part of our salaries to a worthy cause?

Tell us what you want—we'll do it; just give us back our hair!

2

Beginning the Dialogue about Hair Loss

My own hair loss began while I was in high school during the 1960s. Long, straight hair was in vogue and my thick, full-bodied hair and its urge to wave too much was the bane of my existence. I'd spend hours trying to straighten it into the poker-straight styles of the Beatles' girlfriends and the models of the time. I grew up in New York's Hudson Valley, where a hot, humid summer day was enough to send me into fits as my newly ironed hair sprung back to its waves. I ironed my hair far more than I ever ironed my clothes, and my mother blamed the constant straightening for the thinning of my hair, which began in my late teens.

I'll never forget the words written to me in a high school note: "and you're going bald, too." The words before that had something to do with my hips, and the entire note revolved around some now long-forgotten argument, but the words "going bald" left me shaken.

At around age nineteen, I lost a lot of weight in a short period of time due to crash dieting and my hair loss worsened. I know now that while these factors may have aggravated and contributed to my hair loss, stopping the ironing and eating a good diet wouldn't necessarily have resulted in my hair turning around. Likely, they were simply "triggers" that helped bring my female pattern hair loss (genetic hair loss) to the fore.

While my hair loss did not progress quickly through my thirties and forties, now that I'm in my fifties, I believe it's getting noticeably thinner. And while I would mention my thinning pate with various doctors I saw, they didn't say much about it, and it became more of an embarrassment to continually bring it up than to simply ignore it. Physical exams never uncovered any illness that could be causing the hair loss, and since baldness ran in my family, I became resigned to my fate.

My story is not isolated, and judging from the women who have contacted me, I would say mine is far from the worst case of hair loss.

Some of these women's stories are heart-wrenching with despair, while others are from women who heroically embrace their baldness. Nonetheless, whether they are in the early stages of thinning or dealing with frank baldness, they speak openly about how their hair loss affects their self-esteem and their lives and echo the one overriding theme—frustration with finding the causes of their hair loss and coping with it on a daily basis.

Some of the women have given me permission to use their names; others asked that I use a pseudonym, a request I've respected.

Losing Our Hair, Losing Our Minds

Virginia is a seventeen-year-old high school senior whose hair loss began when she was five years old. She suffers from alopecia areata (AA). She says she quit going to the doctor because the steroid injections into her scalp were painful and expensive, and she got to the point where she gave up hope. AA, which is believed to be an autoimmune disorder, will often come and go over the years, sometimes resolving on its own.

"I'm only seventeen, so I'd have to say [my hair loss] affects every waking second of my life. Two years ago, over a course of about eight months, I lost all my hair. I was put on antidepressants and I tried to commit suicide," Virginia writes. She says that she ended up hating everyone around her, and she especially resented it when people would ask her questions about her hair. "I stopped caring about who I was or what I did to myself. I started to do drugs and drink alcohol until it made me sick."

Virginia's hair has now grown in enough to nearly cover most of her bald spots. "But I constantly have [bald spots] appearing and then growing in and then reappearing," she says, adding that she is always monitoring how much hair is falling out and worries constantly that she will be bald again. Such obsession is common in women dealing with hair loss.

Moreover, since the episode in which she lost all her hair, Virginia says she cannot stand to have people touch her head. "I also can't stand the feeling of hair on my body, because it reminds me that my hair is falling out."

Paula's hair has always been thin. Two years ago, at age forty-six, she had fibroid tumors removed and ended up losing most of her hair, but her doctors told her that it would grow back. It hasn't.

"I wear a wig all the time," Paula says. While tests ruled out any underlying physical cause for her hair loss, other than the trauma of the operation, she mentions that she did lose a lot of blood due to heavy menstrual cycles through the years. "My hair is thin all over my head," she says. "I keep it covered all the time with a wig or a hat. I am too embarrassed to even go to a hairdresser to get the little I have left cut. I would like to know where would I go next for help. What kind of doctor should I see?"

Lauren, fifty, a thyroid cancer survivor, noticed her hair was beginning to thin about two years ago, but normal lab tests did not turn up anything. Finally, it was revealed that her thyroid medication was causing elevated levels of the thyroid hormone. "I was elated to think this was the problem, but after six months of being on a lower dose and my levels [returning] to normal, my condition is still the same," she says.

She is devastated by her hair loss. "My life is over, essentially. My love life is gone. I was a very attractive woman with bouncy hair that I could wrap up in a huge clip and look gorgeous," Lauren writes. Now she cries when she tries to style her hair and when she sweeps up the hair from the floor.

"I see myself as a dandelion. One good gust of wind and it will all blow away. I feel like I'm dying," she says.

Angela, thirty-five, is a special education teacher whose hair thinned severely on the top of her head and at the temples by her last year of college. "I'm conscious that others are always staring at my hair and scalp," she says. "I may look into a wig. Where I am, hair is a real big deal, and you can't have 'see-through' hair. I've had many strangers ask what happened to my hair, so I know I need a wig." Many of the parents at the school where she works have approached her and asked if there is anything wrong.

"I was a competitive swimmer until my last year of college. I stopped because of my hair, which was the end of a dream. So this [hair loss] is life-limiting. I'm tired of explaining that I'm not sick, that my hair loss is not my fault," Angela told me.

Angela says she rarely dates anymore, as so much of her day is consumed covering the bald areas. "I'm tired of it all," she says. "I also resent people who say there's a cure, because there isn't, no medicine has slowed my hair loss. I wonder what my head will look like by the time I'm forty!"

Tina, fifty, puts her battle with hair loss succinctly. She says that her self-image is getting worse each day.

"[I'm] losing my connection with myself. Losing my identity. Losing my mind over this," Tina says.

She believes that stress has been the trigger for her hair loss, as her hair began falling out after the deaths of her parents and a diagnosis of rheumatoid arthritis. "I know it sounds superficial, but my hair has always been the feature that helped me feel feminine and attractive, since I never considered myself to be a great looker."

Along with feeling unattractive and unfeminine, there are other common themes and questions in the responses the women have sent to me.

Finding help has proved frustrating to most women. While it's easy to say hair loss isn't a life-threatening disease, reading through the responses to my survey leads me to wonder if the side effects of hair loss—depression, low self-esteem, thoughts of suicide—might point to a condition more serious than what some label as simply a cosmetic issue. The majority of women answering my questionnaire have little faith in the medical profession.

Many of them have spent thousands of dollars seeking medical testing and treatment. Some have even gone to the top hair-loss specialists in the country and still do not know a definitive reason for their hair loss.

While many women have been given diagnoses, among the most frustrated were those diagnosed with female pattern hair loss (FPHL), because, unfortunately, the medical profession has little to offer them. And I sense from their replies that it wasn't so much the diagnosis that left these women feeling abandoned, but it was the perception that their condition was not taken seriously. They say that they feel that many avenues of possible diagnosis and treatment were left unexplored. Moreover, they feel that the medical profession was insensitive to the psychological distress the condition causes them.

While someone not suffering from hair loss might not understand this, for a woman whose hair is diminishing daily, hair—the lack of it, or trying to regrow it—is a daily obsession. It's not something she can put aside.

A rainy or windy day becomes a styling obstacle; an outing to the beach or being in bright sunlight where her scalp might more noticeably show through her hair is a challenge to her self-confidence; meeting new people, going on a job interview, and dating are difficult at best. One young woman who wears a wig says she isn't sure when in a new relationship she should broach the subject of her hair loss.

When a woman is dealing with hair loss and everything she has tried appears to be failing her, she will continue the search. She will buy any snake oil preparation available, and she will latch onto any hope, any promise of a cure someone makes. The unfortunate consequence of this is that a woman may simply be throwing good money after bad hair solutions, and worse, she may be actually making her condition worse or jeopardizing her health.

"This is a strange situation. I don't think any woman thinks she will lose her hair, especially when she is still fairly young, and so quickly that you almost can't adjust to it," Cindy, fifty-three, another woman suffering with alopecia areata, told me. She says she has always been healthy—exercised, watched her weight, and had thick, healthy hair up to the time when it just began falling out in patches. "This is the last thing I ever thought would happen to me," she says. "I would have expected cancer before I would have thought about this, and I know that may sound strange, but it is the truth."

Sara, twenty-seven, told me that she thinks about her hair loss every day. "I absolutely hate it. I get angry, depressed, frustrated," she says.

For Melissa, twenty, dealing with her hair loss has been "emotional hell," but she notes that as she learns to deal with it, it is getting better. Learning to cope, what to do, and what solutions are available is indeed helpful, but Melissa adds, "I hate always worrying about it. That's what bothers me most. I feel like I waste a lot of time and energy on my hair. I just wish I didn't have to think about it."

These are among the most common questions the women answering my survey asked me:

- What is causing my hair loss? Will it grow back?
- Is my hair loss a symptom of disease?
- I had silicone breast implants; could they be affecting my hair loss?
- My doctor doesn't listen to me; how do I find Dr. Right?
- Are there medical treatments for my type of hair loss? How safe are they?
- Will modifying my diet help?
- Do vitamins, herbs, minerals, and other dietary supplements help stop hair loss?
- Could the medications, vitamins, herbs, or minerals I'm taking be causing my hair loss?
- I'm resigned to living with my hair loss. How do I choose a wig, hair additions, extensions, or other hair prostheses?
- How do I explain my hair loss to other people?
- What is the latest research? Are we any closer to hair cloning?

I will try to shed light on these and other questions concerning women's hair loss. Unlike a lot of other books and experts, I am not going to promise you a cure or even outline a treatment plan. There may not be one for you right now, but the future may hold a cure for all of us, and I hope the information provided in this book will give you the tools to find the best option for you at this moment and prevent you from spending time and money traveling the wrong path. Mostly, I hope breaking the silence on this taboo will yield a greater interest in finding better treatments or the elusive cure.

Trying to Outfox the Fox

"Alopecia" is the general term for baldness. The original Greek word means "fox"; its English usage alludes to the patchy baldness seen in the animals when they suffer from mange. But to me this seems a fitting derivation for the name of a condition with a cause that is often mysterious, usually cunning, and always frustrating.

Understanding the way hair grows will help you understand the diagnosis and treatment of your hair loss. It will also serve as a guide for discussing your hair loss with your physician as he or she takes steps to diagnose your particular condition.

There are about 150,000 hair follicles on the typical head, and each produces and sheds a single hair in a cyclic fashion. The most active phase is the growth, or anagen, phase. At any one time, about 85 to 90 percent of the hair on your head is in the anagen phase, growing on average about a half-inch each month, or six inches per year, although medical and other factors can affect this growth rate. The anagen stage lasts from six to ten years.

Catagen, the next stage, is a period of transition, affecting about 2 to 3 percent of scalp follicles at any one time. During this period of controlled regression, hair stops growing.

Normally, the hairs found in your hairbrush or the sink are there as a result of the telogen stage, because it is during this stage that the hair fiber is easily pulled out through combing, brushing, or shampooing. About 10 to

15 percent of your hair is in this resting stage, and it lasts from thirty to ninety days. After the telogen stage, the hair growth cycle begins again, returning to the active anagen phase.

Hair loss can occur when a hair follicle is prematurely pushed into the telogen phase or when any of the other stages are interrupted for some reason.

It is normal to shed about 50 to 150 hairs a day, but when the rate of hair fall exceeds the rate of regrowth, or if the new hair shafts are thinner or hair falls out in patches, thinning or baldness occurs. Hair loss may be temporary or permanent.

The signs of hair loss include:

- Decreased ponytail diameter
- More hair than usual in shower drain, on pillow, or in brush
- Hair on the top of the head is shorter than the rest, or thinning in the center part of the head is widening, or there is a diffuse thinning over the entire top of the head. Diffuse hair loss means that the hair is thinning all over the head, not just in a specific area or areas.

According to many medical experts, by the time there is a visible sign of hair loss, you have probably lost as much as 40 to 50 percent of your hair, which makes finding the cause of your hair loss sooner rather than later paramount.

3

The Many Causes of Hair Loss

If hair loss could be traced to one cause, treating and curing it would be easy. Unfortunately, that is not the case. An underlying health problem, fungal infections, genetic propensities, or a myriad of other things could all be contributing to your hair loss.

Is Something Wrong with Me?
Hair Loss as a Symptom of Disease

Hair loss may be a symptom of a disease and not an end diagnosis in itself. In terms of your overall health, ruling out an underlying condition that may be causing your hair loss is important. This is where self-diagnosis can, at best, lead you down the wrong path and waste precious time and money; at worst, it can endanger your health.

Diagnostic tests are required to determine if your hair loss is caused or triggered by an ongoing disease process. Sometimes, even after a disease such as hypothyroidism is treated, hair loss may continue. Nonetheless, stabilizing

Hair Loss Myth #1

If your mother's brothers are bald, you may inherit the trait.

Not true, but many people still believe. Don't blame your mom alone for this one. You inherit hair loss from both parents. Moreover, it is not a recessive trait like blue eyes, where you would need to inherit a copy from both parents. Researchers believe that if either your mother or father has hair loss, you have a 50 percent chance of inheriting it! (See FPHL on page 35.)

—*Anita Bhorjee*

the disorder is important before proper treatment of your hair loss can begin.

Systemic lupus erythematosus (SLE), hyper/hypothyroidism, and polycystic ovary syndrome (PCOS) are among the diseases that may be associated with thinning hair.

Lupus

SLE (also known as lupus) is a serious systemic condition categorized as an autoimmune disorder that may affect many organ systems, including the skin, joints, and internal organs. An autoimmune disorder occurs when the body's own immune system attacks the body.

The symptoms of lupus include a telltale "butterfly rash" over the nose and cheeks, joint pain, kidney problems, muscle disorders, and swollen glands. Hair loss occurs in about 50 percent of patients with lupus and, according to an article in *Cosmetic Surgery Times*, is marked by short frontal hairs.

Thyroid Problems

Hypothyroidism, or underactive thyroid, is a condition in which the thyroid doesn't produce enough thyroid hormones. Some of the disease's symptoms include hair loss, thin or brittle hair and nails, fatigue, weakness, cold intolerance, unexplained weight gain, depression, and joint or muscle pain.

Hyperthyroidism, or overactive thyroid, is the opposite of hypothyroidism; it is a metabolic imbalance involving an overproduction of thyroid hormones. The usual symptoms include weight loss, increased appetite, nervousness, restlessness, heat intolerance, increased sweating, and fatigue. Hair loss may also be present.

Both hypothyroidism and hyperthyroidism can be marked by sudden hair loss, and, according to an article in Prevention, may be marked by more diffuse thinning at the front of the hairline or on the crown.

Polycystic Ovary Syndrome (PCOS)

PCOS accounts for about 80 to 90 percent of androgen disorders in women. An androgen disorder means that male hormones, such as testosterone, are present in either too great or too little quantity.

Hair loss or thinning in what is usually considered a male pattern—at temples and crown—is one of the heralding features of this disease, but an overall thinning can signal its presence as well. In addition, other symptoms go hand in hand with PCOS: chronic irregular menstrual cycles or absent periods, infertility or difficulty conceiving because of non-ovulation, obesity, sudden unexplained weight gain, adult acne, hirsutism (excessive hair growth), and type 2 diabetes or insulin resistance.

In her book *Living with PCOS* Angela Boss cites this statistic: It is estimated that from 5 to 10 percent of all women are affected by PCOS, which translates to five to ten million women in the United States alone, and it affects women of all ages, from adolescence to menopause.

It is important to understand that PCOS, like thyroid disease and many other disorders associated with hair loss, affects the endocrine system, which produces and regulates the body's hormones.

Other Endocrine Disorders

Ferreting out a possible endocrine disorder, however mild, could be crucial to getting an accurate diagnosis and potential cure for your hair loss. Other endocrine disorders for which hair loss may be a symptom include diabetes, Hashimoto's disease (thyroiditis), hypopituitarism, and hypothalamic disorders.

Nonendocrine Disorders

Nonendocrine disorders may also have hair loss as a symptom: liver disease, inflammatory bowel diseases such as Crohn's disease, syphilis, liver and kidney failure, candida (yeast infection), and certain cancers such as Hodgkin's lymphoma and leukemia.

Naturally, if you have a really serious disease, hair loss will not be your only symptom, but it could be among your first symptoms, so getting a proper workup to ensure that your hair loss does not have a physical cause is your first step in your search for a solution.

Is My Medication Causing My Hair Loss?

Drug-Induced Alopecia

While an underlying disease may trigger hair loss, many medications, both prescription and nonprescription, are implicated in the condition. "Drug-induced alopecia usually involves pharmaceutical alteration of the cycling process [the phases of hair growth]," writes Jerry Shapiro, M.D., author of *Hair Loss: Principles of Diagnosis and Management of Alopecia,* a definitive text on hair loss.

The anagen or telogen phase may be altered with the use of some medications, and the alopecias that result are often grouped under anagen effluvium (AE) and telogen effluvium (TE).

In listing the drugs that may be associated with hair loss, which I've culled from Shapiro's text, I've put the brand name of the drug in parentheses, if available. Where a drug has more than one brand name, I've tried to include the most common.

WARNING: Do not stop any prescribed medication without first speaking to your doctor.

Anagen Effluvium

Usually when one thinks of hair loss associated with drugs, chemotherapy—a cancer treatment—comes to mind. Some drugs used in chemotherapy cause hair loss in almost 100 percent of the patients given them, and the hair loss can be partial or total, which is the bad news. The good news is that anagen effluvium is usually completely reversible.

The most common drugs used to treat cancer that cause hair loss include:

- Doxorubicin (Adriamycin)
- Cyclophosphamide (Cytoxan)

- Methotrexate (This drug is also used as a treatment for rheumatoid arthritis.)
- Fluorouracil (5-FU)
- Vincristine (Oncovin)
- Daunorubicin (Cerubidine)
- Bleomycin (Blenoxane)
- Hydroxycarbamide (formerly hydroxyurea)

Some drugs used in combination chemotherapy (treatment with more than one drug at a time in what is sometimes called a "cocktail") may also exacerbate AE. These include:

- Chlorambucil (Leukeran)
- Thiotepa (Thioplex)
- Cytarabine (Ara-C)
- Vinblastine (Velban)
- Dactinomycin (Actinomycin)

Telogen Effluvium

Shapiro lists more than two hundred medications in his text that may be associated with drug-induced telogen effluvium. While for most people taking these drugs, their hair remains unaffected, if you are on any of these medications and your hair loss began shortly after starting treatment, mention it to your doctor.
These include:

- Anticoagulants such as heparin (Calciparine) and warfarin (Coumadin). May be dose-related.
- Anti-thyroid drugs such as iodine, methylthiouracil, propylthiouracil, and carbimazole (Remember: thyroid disease itself may cause hair loss, so keep this in mind when undergoing treatment.)

- Lithium, used to treat bipolar disorder, may affect thyroid function, which should be monitored in patients taking the drug, and in turn affect hair growth.
- Tricyclic antidepressants such as amitriptyline (Elavil), amoxapine (Asendin), desipramine (Norpramin), doxepin (Adapin), and nortriptyline (Aventyl)
- Tetracyclic antidepressants such as maprotiline (Ludiomil) and trazodone (Desyrel)
- Selective serotonin reuptake inhibitors (SSRIs) such as fluoxetine (Prozac), sertraline (Zoloft), and paroxetine (Paxil) have only a rare association with hair loss (see below).
- Treatments for high blood pressure—beta-blockers such as Inderal and Lopressor, the ACE (angiotensin converting enzyme) inhibitor Captopril (Capoten)
- Interferons
- Acne treatments Soriatane and Accutane
- Statin drugs (for lowering cholesterol) atorvastatin (Lipitor), cerivastatin (Baycol—no longer on the market), simvastatin (Zocor), and pravastatin (Pravachol), as well as the SSRI antidepressant/smoking cessation aid bupropion (Wellbutrin/Zyban)

In his text Shapiro mentions that SSRI-induced alopecia progresses according to what he calls "a typical pattern of reversible diffuse alopecia," occurring after two to six months of use, but "sometimes alopecia may develop 1.5 years following fluoxetine introduction." He also cites a case in which alopecia was still evident more than a year after discontinuing the medication.

Nonprescription Drugs May Cause Hair Loss Too

It's not only prescription drugs that may affect your hair; over-the-counter medications can also be associated with hair loss. They include ibuprofen (Motrin, Advil), naproxen (Aleve), acetaminophen (Tylenol), and aspirin. While obviously hair loss associated with pain relievers is rare, if you take these pain relievers on a regular basis or if you noticed that your hair loss began shortly after you started taking them more regularly for chronic pain or another condition, don't rule them out!

Vitamins and other supplements may also be implicated in hair loss, and some may surprise you. Excess intake of vitamins A and E has been associated with hair loss, and it's interesting to note that vitamin A deficiency is also associated with hair loss.

The take-home message in all this is that it is important to tell your physician every prescription or over-the-counter drug, vitamin, and supplement you are taking and when you began taking them. Medications, vitamins, and herbs may not be the main cause of your hair loss, but they could be part of the problem, especially if you noticed your hair loss began or worsened six months or so after you began taking them.

NOTE: The drugs and supplements I've listed are by no means the only medications that may be associated with hair loss. Moreover, there are more and more drugs coming on the market every day, many of which are likely to have hair loss as a side effect. Read package inserts.

Telogen Effluvium (TE)

Besides certain medications, there are a number of other conditions that can interrupt the telogen phase of hair growth. According to most medical sources, the inciting event triggering telogen effluvium—whether a medication or any of the other causes that are listed below, such as a high fever—usually occurs several weeks to several months before hair shedding occurs. Once the offending trigger is found and corrected, hair will usually begin to regrow.

There are two types of telogen effluvium: acute telogen effluvium, in which the hair shedding lasts less than six months, and chronic telogen effluvium, in which it lasts longer than six months. The latter, naturally, can be more difficult to treat, as will be discussed later.

Hair Loss after Childbirth

Postpartum telogen effluvium, or hair shedding after giving birth, is common, albeit particularly disturbing, since often during pregnancy our hair appears to get fuller. In pregnancy, the anagen phase is prolonged, with the percentage of anagen hairs increasing to 84 percent in the first trimester and to 94 percent in the final trimester. About one to four months after giving birth, the hair cycle resumes, and the telogen phase kicks in, resulting in a cascade of seemingly greater-than-usual shedding. This may continue, distressingly, for several months afterward.

When your hair is falling out by handfuls, it's not easy to calmly accept that this is normal, but in most instances, it is. For women who have been dealing with female pattern hair loss (FPHL), however, that episode of thicker hair was a godsend, and its subsequent falling out is like awakening to find there was no prince, there was no ball, and both shoes are intact.

Blood loss, low plasma protein, psycho-physical trauma, and other conditions following childbirth may also aggravate the condition. The good news is that hair usually grows back within a year, and the TE is usually less severe with subsequent pregnancies.

Illness with High Fever, Crash Dieting, and Other Causes of TE

You may notice hair shed within eight to ten weeks after an illness with a high fever or surgery. Crash dieting, anorexia, or bulimia may also result in TE, likely due to a lack of sufficient protein.

However, I was intrigued during my research to come across a reference to a study funded by the Atkins Center for Complementary Medicines, which, along with touting some of the benefits of Atkins's high-protein, high-fat, low-carbohydrate diet, also noted, nearly as an aside, that 10 percent of the people in this particular study experienced hair loss. I list the effect of low-carb diets here with the caveat that this is not well researched yet, and other factors might be implicated in the hair loss noted in the study. Could this finding possibly be due to a lack of folic acid and biotin, since the high-protein diet limits many sources of those nutrients, such as orange juice and whole grains?

Other deficiencies or toxicities associated with hair loss include zinc deficiency, essential fatty acid deficiency, and mercury toxicity. Note, however, that you should not start taking supplements on your own if one of these deficiencies has not been diagnosed or you do not have other symptoms of the deficiency.

For example, if too much zinc is taken—more than 25 milligrams a day—it may adversely affect the absorption of iron, thereby causing or worsening an iron deficiency. Nutrition and supplements will be further discussed later on in the book.

Ferritin Levels

Low iron levels or low ferritin (stored iron) levels are also implicated in TE; however, this area is so controversial that I'm dedicating an entire chapter to it (see chapter 8).

Hormone Supplements and Birth-Control Pills

Hormones and women's hair loss are another controversial area. Starting, changing, or stopping birth-control pills can affect your hair. They can be implicated in TE and also in FPHL, both as a cause and as a cure. Some women experience TE after stopping birth-control pills, similar to what is seen in postpartum hair loss. This is seen less with low-dose contraceptive pills. While some doctors will prescribe birth-control pills as a treatment for hair loss, keep in mind that studies show mixed results with their use. The role hormones play in women's hair loss will also be discussed later.

Possible Causes of Hair Loss You Might Not Suspect

Then there are some rather surprising and unusual potential causes of hair loss that I came across in my research. As you continue reading here, keep in mind there may be other strange things that could be implicated in your particular case of hair loss. As will be emphasized later on in this book, you need to be a good detective and have a doctor willing to be your partner in the investigation, especially if your hair loss begins suddenly and there are no bald or balding people in your family history.

Silicone Breast Implants

One woman asked me if her silicone breast implants might have caused her hair loss. I nearly dismissed the question, until I did a Google search and found the FDA's 1995 document titled "A Status Report on Breast Implant Safety." Breast implants have been on the market since the early 1960s, almost twenty years before the enactment of the first medical device law in 1976, which put their regulation under FDA auspices. After widespread reports of adverse reactions to silicone gel–filled breast implants and a lack of evidence supporting their safe use, the FDA ordered them off the market in April 1992. Silicone breast implants have been associated with the possible development of "autoimmune-like" disorders, and among the listed symptoms is "unusual hair loss."

I also found three studies listed in PubMed, the database associated with the U.S. National Library of Medicine, discussing this relationship. One study discussed what was dubbed a "multiple sclerosis–like syndrome" associated with silicone gel breast implants. Out of the twenty-six women in the study, twelve had hair loss.

Another study of eighty-seven patients with breast implants found that 13 percent of the women experienced hair loss, and the third study of three hundred women included hair loss in a list of "miscellaneous conditions."

NOTE: At the time of the writing of this book, an FDA advisory committee recommended that the agency allow silicone breast implants back on the market.

Face-lifts and Hair Loss

Now this seems just cruel. It is estimated that temporal hair loss occurs in just over 8 percent of patients who undergo rhytidectomy, or face lift, according to a study presented at the sixtieth annual meeting of the American Academy of Dermatology. Lead researcher of the study, Cindy Y. Li, D.O., quoted in an article in *Dermatology Times*, explains: "Commonly, after a face-lift procedure, due to a lot of undermining of the skin and a lot of manipulation of the skin, the hair follicles are sometimes temporarily traumatized, and as a result, there may be temporary hair loss in the area where the procedure was done." Although the hair typically regrows, she does note that in some cases the loss may be permanent. She and her colleagues at the University of California, Los Angeles, recommend the use of topical minoxidil for this problem.

While the incidence among such patients is rare, if you already suffer from hair loss, measures such as using topical minoxidil to prevent the acute TE that sometimes accompanies rhytidectomy should be taken.

Alopecia Areata

Alopecia areata is a type of hair loss that can strike without warning and is marked by round or oval patches completely devoid of hair that may be found on the scalp or any hair-bearing part of the body.

It is thought to be an autoimmune disorder caused by lymphocytes surrounding the hair follicle, leading to abnormal differentiation and breakage of the growing hair.

According to the National Alopecia Areata Foundation (NAAF), alopecia areata is estimated to affect 2 percent, or four million people in the United States, and while it strikes people of all ages and both sexes, about 60 percent of the people suffering with the condition are under twenty.

In contrast to patients who suffer from telogen effluvium, which, as previously mentioned, may be triggered by an underlying condition, people who experience alopecia areata are basically healthy. However, they may be prone to other conditions; they do appear to have an increased incidence of thyroiditis and allergies, research shows. "Alopecia areata often occurs in families whose members have had asthma, hay fever, atopic eczema, or other autoimmune diseases such as thyroid disease, early onset diabetes, rheumatoid arthritis, lupus erythematosus, vitiligo, pernicious anemia, or Addison's disease," according to the NAAF.

In most cases of alopecia areata, hair will regrow without treatment within one year. However, 7 to 10 percent of patients have a severe chronic form of the condition, with complete loss of hair on the head (alopecia totalis) or loss of hair over the entire body (alopecia universalis).

According to the NAAF, it is not known whether something outside the body, such as a virus, triggers the autoimmune response, or whether it is initiated by the body itself. Moreover, Madeleine Duvic, M.D., chief of dermatology at M. D. Anderson's Melanoma and Skin Center, who is leading research in alopecia areata, said that the trigger does not have to be the same in each patient. "Our studies have shown that only half of identical twins will have alopecia areata, suggesting an environmental factor is as important as genes," she told me during an interview.

However, the foundation says recent research suggests some people have genetic markers that appear to increase their susceptibility to the condition and that determine how severe it will be when it strikes. The condition is believed to be hereditary, with about 20 percent of those with it having someone else in the family who also suffers from the condition. However, if alopecia areata first strikes after age thirty-five, it is less likely another family member will have it.

Research conducted by Duvic and her colleagues also suggests that alopecia areata may be triggered by environmental factors, such as viruses, but these differ from person to person. Viruses that have been associated with this type of hair loss include cytomegalovirus and hepatitis C. Drugs such as haloperidol, rifampin, and zotepine have also been implicated.

Alopecia areata may be the most cunning and fox-like of all the various forms of hair loss, because while the condition strikes people who are otherwise healthy and is not medically disabling, for many, especially the very young, it is a devastating condition. It is sly like a fox in its sudden onset and sometimes equally sudden remission. Even after years of hair loss, the condition can mysteriously disappear, but it can also, just as mysteriously, reappear, which leaves its sufferers ever wary and anticipating its possible return.

There is no known cure for alopecia areata, but there are treatments that may help (see chapter 6).

Researchers, led by Duvic, are undertaking a study of alopecia areata and gathering information in a registry sponsored by the National Institute of Arthritis and Musculoskeletal and Skin Diseases (NIAMS), a division of the National Institutes of Health. The purpose of the study, which is being conducted at five research centers across the United States, is to collect patient information and blood samples from people with alopecia areata for further research. To register or find out more about the ongoing research, visit www.alopeciaareataregistry.org.

Hair Pulling and Other Types of Hair Loss

Along with interruptions of the hair-growth cycle, other types of hair loss can be brought about by trauma to the scalp or various fungal infections. Some of these conditions are extremely rare and will not be the main focus of this book. However, these types of hair loss should be on your doctor's radar if your case does not appear to fall into one of the more common categories.

Trichtotillomania

This type of hair loss, also known as chronic hair-pulling or morbid hair-pulling, is considered a psychological disorder, as it is self-induced. The hair loss results from the person deliberately pulling out his or her own hair, and the pattern of hair loss results in a typical "monk's fringe," with the hair in the center of the head pulled out. It is considered a traumatic alopecia. While for children the condition is more often manifested in boys than in girls, among adults, women are the more frequent hair-pullers.

Traction Alopecia

Traction alopecia typically occurs when there is sustained tension on the scalp through styling techniques such as tight ponytails or braiding. Bleaching and straightening can also cause it. Traction alopecia is most often seen in African American women who style their hair in tight braids or who use chemical straighteners. It is also seen in Japanese geisha who attach hairpieces to their hair to create their intricate signature hairstyles.

In traction alopecia, the hair can often sustain the trauma of the tension for awhile, and if the offending practice is stopped, the hair loss can be reversed. However, if the pulling of the hair through severe styling methods continues, the hair follicle will stop producing hair.

Cicatricial or Scarring Alopecias

Cicatricial alopecias are categorized as either inflammatory or noninflammatory and represent a group of diseases that are characterized by a lack of follicular ostia (pores).

Inflammatory cicatricial alopecias include chronic cutaneous lupus erythematosus (CCLE), lichen planopilaris (LPP), and folliculitis decalvans (FD). Some types of noninflammatory scarring alopecias are pseudopelade of Brocq (PP) and follicular degeneration syndrome. CCLE, LPP, and PP are the most common scarring alopecias.

An interesting note appears in Shapiro's text: "Pelade is the French word for alopecia areata. Pseudopelade

Hair Loss Myth #2

Hair loss is normal in men, but abnormal in women.

Not true. Most men and women who lose their hair to pattern baldness are perfectly healthy. The American Academy of Dermatology estimates that of the thirty million American women who lose their hair, 70 percent of them have female pattern hair loss.

—*Anita Bhorjee*

refers to 'like alopecia areata but not alopecia areata.' In pseudopelade (Brocq), the follicular ostia are not present, while in AA they are most certainly present."

One woman who wrote me from England suffers from pseudopelade of Brocq and is the only person diagnosed with the condition in her county. It is very rare.

Female Pattern Hair Loss (Androgenetic Alopecia)

I've listed this category last, as it accounts for the majority of hair loss seen in women. It affects 20 to 50 percent of women by age fifty, according to the American Academy of Dermatology. Female pattern hair loss is considered hereditary, although the exact inheritance pattern is debated. If baldness runs in your family, on either your mother's or your father's side, there is a good chance you will have some hair thinning or frank hair loss.

While the condition is often referred to as androgenetic alopecia (AGA), I have chosen to primarily use the term "female pattern hair loss" (FPHL) to describe it, as current research is showing that this is not just the female version of male pattern baldness, and experts in the field of hair loss research are now using FPHL to describe the process in women.

Research into FPHL is still evolving, and most of what we know comes from the study of pattern baldness in men. An enzyme (proteins that facilitate chemical reactions), 5 alpha-reductase, is involved in setting the stage for pattern baldness. This enzyme is responsible for converting testosterone into dihydrotestosterone (DHT). DHT attaches to the androgen (male sex hormone) receptor in hair follicles, and in people who have the genes for genetic balding, the cascade is triggered, the hair follicles become progressively miniaturized, and hair loss occurs.

Androgen receptor protein levels are 30 percent greater in balding frontal hair follicles than in occipital (back of the head) areas in both men and women, with women having 40 percent less total receptor content than men, Shapiro notes. This means the balding usually occurs in a pattern, with the back of the head typically retaining more, or a nearly normal amount of hair, as opposed to diffuse or overall thinning.

Another enzyme comes into play as well, and this one may hold some hope for future research, particularly in women—the cytochrome P450 aromatase enzyme. This enzyme is also involved in the metabolism or conversion of androgens, but instead of converting testosterone to DHT, it converts testosterone to estradiol and estrone, two forms of the female sex hormone estrogen. "Aromatase is significantly higher in the hair follicles of women," Shapiro writes in his text, and thus it helps to explain why women with FPHL "usually retain their frontal hairline and usually have less loss than men with [androgenetic alopecia]."

Researchers are uncertain about the role that estrogen plays in hair growth and whether the estrogens formed from aromatase act to suppress the severity of hair loss for women or help suppress the overall load of androgens formed at the hair follicle. I personally believe that this area holds a lot of promise for possible future research. If aromatase helps retain estrogen in the hair follicles, perhaps if it could somehow be bolstered, it might protect the hair follicles from attack by DHT.

Female pattern hair loss, which can start as early as puberty, usually progresses gradually, although there can be triggering factors such as hormonal changes, including starting and stopping birth-control pills and postpartum, peri-menopausal, and postmenopausal states,

Hair Loss Myth #3

Hats cause hair loss.

A hundred years ago, before the revelation in the 1940s that hair loss was linked to genes and androgens, any reputable doctor would have informed you of the obvious cause of your hair loss—hats! This conclusion was reached after noting that men lost hair in the area of the scalp covered by their hats. The doctors of the day opined that the hats restricted key arteries of the scalp, notes Kerry Segrave in his book, *Baldness: A Social History.* Women, it was thought, fared better because of their softer, looser-fitting chapeaux. This myth overlaps another that exists to this day—that decreased circulation leads to thinning hair.

—*Anita Bhorjee*

Shapiro says. "These events, which can elicit a telogen effluvium, may unmask a tendency for AGA," he explains in his text. He also says that hyperandrogenism (an over-production of androgen) needs to be determined—such as is found with polycystic ovary syndrome—and notes that SAHA syndrome (seborrhea, alopecia, hirsutism, and acne) is a hallmark for androgen excess in female patients. He adds that for the vast majority of women with FPHL, this is not the problem.

Because it has been observed that the androgen-to-hair-loss connection is not as clear-cut in women as in men, some researchers have proposed four subsets of female pattern hair loss:

- Early onset with androgen excess
- Early onset without androgen excess
- Late onset/postmenopausal with androgen excess
- Late onset/postmenopausal without androgen excess

What this means is that women may or may not have androgen excess, or abnormal levels of circulating androgens, but they may still manifest a pattern type of baldness. This may also help explain why some medical treatments that work so well for men only work in a small percentage of women. We are different!

Female pattern hair loss can be exceedingly frustrating for women to deal with, as it keeps most of us wondering if, and often hoping that, something else is going on that could be cured and thus result in hair regrowth. But unfortunately, this type of hair loss is at best controlled through various treatments and rarely "cured."

Breaking the Silence:
Talking about Hair Loss

"I want to get a clearly defined cause for my hair loss, as not knowing why for seven years feels as helpless and frustrating as the hair loss itself," Barbara, fifty-three, told me.

She says she is not satisfied with the reasons she's so far been given for her hair loss. And why should she be? She consulted several doctors and received a different diagnosis from each one.

Barbara and many of the other women who wrote to me say they don't believe doctors perform enough tests to try to find a cause for their hair loss because it is viewed mostly as a cosmetic issue or not a terribly important health concern, and therefore they look no further than the scalp—if they even look at the scalp.

Barbara has a lot of underlying physical problems, including having had a hysterectomy. She is questioning if there are possible hormonal imbalances related to her surgery that could be affecting her hair. She also would like her thyroid tested. Barbara is typical of the many women who wrote to me who do not feel that conditions that may be contributing to their hair loss have been ruled out.

Bernice, thirty-three, first noticed her hair thinning at age nineteen but didn't seek medical attention until recently. She has seen many doctors, including her primary care doctor, an endocrinologist, and three dermatologists. The tests that were run showed her iron and thyroid hormone levels were borderline, but she says none of the doctors seemed interested enough to follow through with more tests or to explore her situation further. One of the dermatologists "took one look at my current hair loss pattern, refused to do blood work, handed me a pamphlet on hair loss and a box of topical minoxidil (Rogaine), and said to thank my father for the genes."

Bernice is concerned that the doctors are not listening to her or taking into account her other symptoms, which include long menstrual periods, with only two weeks in between, and hair loss over her entire body, not just on her head. "I want answers about my symptoms and my hair loss. I want the doctor to listen to me," she says.

Cindy, fifty-three, feels "used and abused" by one dermatologist who treated her alopecia areata for two years with a number of treatments—including painful cortisone shots to the scalp—which helped for a while, but after they stopped working, expensive, cosmetic options were suggested "to help my self-esteem."

She feels as if the doctor just wrote her off, and worse, she told me that the doctor she was seeing admonished her for not adhering to the program better! He told her she was not being aggressive enough, and he even claimed that the steroid shots and the topical minoxidil weren't working because of stress. Cindy was left feeling that she was somehow to blame for her hair loss. Stress indeed!

Michelle, forty-one, first began noticing her hair loss in her mid-twenties. Her story is similar to many others. The diagnosis of the cause was not clear, with one doctor's opinion contradicting another's. She has been left with little confidence that there is medical help for her increasingly thinning hair.

Barbara, Bernice, Cindy, and Michelle exemplify the level of frustration the women who write to me have experienced with the medical profession. Their stories are not isolated, and I could fill this book with similar tales. One thing, however, is clear: Finding out why hair loss is occurring is difficult at best, and at worst, many women who are given a definitive diagnosis are not convinced the diagnosis is correct.

Because hair loss, especially women's hair loss, is considered a cosmetic issue for the most part, and because the few treatments available do seem to be working "OK"—for men—the issue isn't on the front lines of medical exploration or even thought about much during regular office visits. This needs to change.

The Psychological Impact of Hair Loss

Several studies have documented how hair loss affects a woman's quality of life. Not surprisingly, one study from the Netherlands assessing women with FPHL found that 75 percent of them expressed negative self-esteem, and 50 percent said they experienced social problems. Another study from Toronto that set out to assess their quality of life found that 40 percent of the women were not satisfied with the way their current doctor managed their hair loss.

A more recent study, published in the *British Medical Journal* by Nigel Hunt and Sue McHale, also looked at the psychological impact of alopecia. Their clinical review of thirty-four studies led them to report that not only do the psychological aspects of hair loss need to be taken into account by practitioners, but the efficacy of psychological treatments should be assessed for helping people cope with the disorder. Moreover, they said that physicians who provide treatment that is likely to be ineffective "may do more psychological harm than medical good."

Even the so-called hair loss experts can be low on the sensitivity scale. Several of the women who wrote to me have gone to some of the top hair loss specialists in the country and are still frustrated. One woman told me she feels she was given the researcher's "cure du jour." She didn't feel she was looked at as an individual but rather as another peg to be plugged into the current theory and treatment the researcher was working on.

Are You Buying into a Franchise of False Hope?

Because there is little help for hair loss and few doctors seem to really "get it," it is tempting to excoriate the entire medical profession and put the question of our hair loss outside the realm of normal medicine.

But where, exactly, does that leave us?

In my opinion, if we write off the help we may be able to get from doctors, two things happen:

- We're left with only one alternative: to seek out hair solutions on our own and possibly fall prey to those "hair specialists" who peddle unapproved treatments or continue to aid our quest in tilting at windmills for an elusive cure. These charlatans will certainly have success at growing something, but it will be their bank accounts, not our hair.
- We remain victims—victims of self-help books offering untried "cures" that may have worked for some but won't work for all. When those remedies fail to work for us, we, like Cindy, blame ourselves and continue to think that somehow, something we did or didn't do is at fault.

I'm reminded of the positive thinking movement that cropped up in the 1970s in relationship to cancer and other diseases. The premise was good—love yourself, meditate, don't harbor negative thoughts, and practice visualization to attack the disease attacking your body. It certainly makes sense that disease is dis-ease.

However, cancer, like many other serious illnesses, cannot simply be wished away. While a good attitude, prayer, and meditation have been found to be important in helping maintain a healthful lifestyle and are particularly important to our quality of life, they are not a cure, even though they are likely an important part of the cure.

We certainly know plenty of ornery people who survived cancer—and plenty of saints who died from it.

The same goes for some of the hair loss "cures" out there touted in books or on Web sites that are outside the realm of the mainstream medical profession. These claim that your doctor isn't trained in the disease or condition the book is covering, or worse, that your doctor is somehow holding back important information that only he or she knows, and you just don't know the secret handshake to elicit the information.

Logic dictates that if someone knew how to cure baldness, the remedy wouldn't be a secret shared only with a few or only found by those who happened across the information on a Web site or in a book. A viable treatment that could control, stop, or cure hair loss would be a potentially large cash cow. If there was a treatment that worked effectively for everyone, we'd all be only too happy to beg, borrow, or steal the money to pay for it. The sad part is, when books or Web sites tout a particular remedy based on anecdotal or personal evidence that is not well documented, we part with our money, hoping it will work for us too.

Buying into a franchise of false hope is isolating; it puts a barrier between us and real treatments that may help. It keeps hair loss in the closet—keeping us silent and ashamed. That said, I'm not going to let the medical profession off the hook.

Talking about the Elephant in the Room

Bring up your hair loss with every doctor you see—the earlier the cause of your hair loss is diagnosed, the better the chance for treatment. Furthermore, it is important that every physician you see understands the distress your hair loss is causing you. Moreover, your hair loss or thinning hair should be part of your physician's overall exam and diagnosis.

Look at it this way: If you took a dog with hair loss to the veterinarian, the doctor would run his or her hands over the dog's coat and ask, "How long has your dog's fur been like this?"

Given that hair loss could be an indicator of a disease process going on, of a physical stressor in your life, or of a reaction to a recently started medication, you would think a doctor might ask you, "How long has your hair been thinning?"

While that may seem like a logical question, your doctor more than likely won't ask it. Physicians are often uneasy bringing up what could be a sensitive subject—our weight, our sex lives . . . our hair.

"If a doctor brings it up, a woman will think you're prying or not addressing the issues she wants addressed," Zoe Draelos, M.D., a dermatologist in private practice and a clinical associate professor in the department of dermatology at Wake Forest University School of Medicine in Winston-Salem, North Carolina, told me. "She needs to bring it up with the doctor, as it is unlikely the doctor will bring it up with [her]."

Draelos's observation points out how deeply the issue of women's hair loss is still in the closet. In fact, I don't think it's just in the closet; it's probably in some old, musty, dust-covered storage box that isn't even being considered for a garage sale.

I realize our physicians may be ignoring the problem because they have so little to offer, or worse, may not even be knowledgeable enough to offer what little there is. Sadly, we must draw attention to it.

For us, our hair loss is the elephant in the room. And we cannot let it be ignored!

Rhani, thirty-one, says that because her hair is basically thick—her part just beginning to widen—physicians haven't taken her hair loss seriously. When she has tried to explain to her physicians that she sheds an unusual amount of hair each day, she is often told, "Don't be silly; you have a wonderful head of hair." While they should know better, since hair loss experts say the earlier you seek treatment the better, many doctors may not take you seriously if they do not see frank bald patches or very noticeable thinning. Since hair loss is viewed by many doctors and other professionals as a cosmetic issue, many of us who do try to find the cause early on are seen as sitting on the low end of the self-esteem scale or, worse, as overly vain.

Rhani, who says it is nothing for her to lose more than four hundred hairs a day, told me she found a way to make her doctors sit up and take notice of the elephant.

"I'd gather up my morning's hair fall from the floor, put it in a big plastic bag, and take it with me to the office," she said. "While they may have thought I might be bringing them a month's worth of hair instead of one day's, they had to pay attention to it."

Pictures showing when your hair was thicker could help plead your case as well. Or consider bringing along a friend or family member to your doctor's visit as support to help explain the changes he or she has observed in your hair.

We need to bring our physicians on the team as our expert advocates in our quest to resolve our hair loss, just as we would if we needed help losing weight or coping with diabetes or dealing with some other chronic condition.

5

Building Your Hair Loss Team

Mary Wendel, M.D., who, with her husband, Mark DiStefano, M.D., runs the Women's Hair Loss Center in Worcester and Newton, Massachusetts, wasn't always a hair loss expert.

She began her medical career as an internist. Her husband is a hair transplant surgeon, and over the past several years, more women began coming to him to see if hair transplantation could help their situations.

"What we found fairly early was that a lot of these women may have other issues that are affecting their hair other than genetic hair loss," she told me. "My husband was so involved doing surgery he didn't have time to sit down and really evaluate women coming in, so that's where I started to see them."

Wendel, as do all the other doctors I interviewed for this book, says that the first thing they do is attempt to rule out any underlying medical causes contributing to hair loss. She notes that her background as an internist puts her in a good position for diagnosing such problems, but she also acknowledges, "When I was in primary care, I didn't know much about hair loss." At that time she would have sent someone to a hair loss specialist. But now, based on the women she sees coming through her center, she advocates a team approach.

For instance, Wendel has diagnosed several women with PCOS at the center. "The symptom they notice the most is that their hair is thinning. We treat them very aggressively hormonally and work very closely with their doctor. I think it's very important that they see a sort of team approach—gynecologist, dermatologist, endocrinologist."

You might seek out an endocrinologist when you or your physician suspects that androgen excess, thyroid problems, or other endocrine-related disorders may be involved in your hair loss. "Should every woman with hair loss see an endocrinologist?" I asked Rhoda Cobin, M.D., FACE, clinical professor of medicine at Mount Sinai School of Medicine in New York City. "I think that would be stating it too broadly," Cobin says. But she adds: "Certainly [for] anyone where there is a suggestion of androgen excess, thyroid disease that's not being well-managed, or menopause issues, endocrinologists are certainly the go-to people for a good, thorough analysis of what the data show and what it doesn't show and how that may be applicable to them. I think dermatologists, and I have some good friends who are dermatologists, may not be quite as aware of all the systemic issues for hormone replacement therapy and are not as involved in managing chronic hyperandrogenetic disorders."

Wendel notes that if you are sent to a specialist, he or she needs to be persistent in finding the underlying cause of your hair loss. She suggests that you find someone who is a specialist in hair loss "and doesn't minimize it and say, 'Oh, well, there's nothing you can do.'"

Finding Dr. Right

Rhani told me that if her dermatologist had explained that with her chronic telogen effluvium she would likely not lose more than 25 to 40 percent of her hair, and that hair loss isn't really visible until 50 percent is lost, it would have helped. "These are very rational talking points," she says. "While I don't know if I would have believed it, it would have certainly been something to cling to. I really just thought my chances for love were over; I thought my life was basically over."

Rhani did not find Dr. Right until she did her own research, even to the point of writing down her findings in what became a small book on the subject. Armed with information, she went to an endocrinologist and asked to try spironolactone for her hair loss, which appears to be working for her.

Cindy found Dr. Right nearly by accident.

She was in a wig store, contemplating the purchase of a wig. While there, leafing through a coupon book, she saw an offer for a facial and decided that rather than make the wig decision right then and there, she would go have a facial. As she removed her ubiquitous baseball cap for the facial, the aesthetician mentioned that one of her clients went to a doctor at UCLA who was using an experimental treatment for alopecia areata, and she gave Cindy the client's number. "That was the most wonderful phone call of my life," she told me.

Wilma, forty-one, searched for three years and sought help from five or six dermatologists before she got help for her chronic telogen effluvium. "Finding a good doctor just completely turned everything around—no matter what the diagnosis had turned out to be. It just made a huge difference finding someone who would listen to me, perform every test available, and then provide treatment," she says.

Silence Is Not Golden

If we haven't told our doctors that this is absolutely devastating to us emotionally and spiritually, we can't expect they will volunteer a shoulder.

Television's pop-psychology guru Dr. Phil often says, "You teach people how to treat you." If we do not explain how this condition affects us, if we keep the silence, silence will surround us. Here's the deal.

Even in cases in which hair loss is hereditary and there is not yet a magic bullet, there are steps that can be taken to preserve the hair you have. You need a partner to see you through this, one you feel confident seeing, who will help you come to terms with what you can and cannot do about your own situation.

Cobin explained that part of being a good physician is that "after doing the evaluation and managing what you can manage, after making sure there is no systemic cause, then you have to just be a good resource for that patient."

A Slow, Gentle Process

On our part, we need to be patient with the process—not an easy task. Are you like me? When I start a new diet, I expect to see instant results, and when I begin a new hair loss treatment, I expect to see a sudden transformation. But unrealistic expectations only lead to disappointment in many aspects of our lives, and hair loss is no different.

Robert S. Haber, M.D., a dermatologist in private practice and an assistant professor of dermatology and pediatrics at Case Western Reserve University School of Medicine in Cleveland, Ohio, told me that the process of diagnosing and treating a woman with hair loss will take close to a year. Because of the hair growth cycle, it will take at least three to six months to see if something is working. "If I can stop the hair loss tomorrow, you're not going to see any significant hair growth for a while. So I'll

Who Is Dr. Right for You?

- Dr. Right is a partner, someone sensitive to the issues surrounding women's hair loss and not just to the clinical aspects of the condition.
- Dr. Right is experienced in treating women's hair loss. Your primary care physician may be able to help direct you, but you may also have to do your own research.
- Dr. Right is someone with whom you will feel a rapport. And when you finally have your answer, you will be satisfied that no stone was left unturned in finding it.

see a person roughly every three months; I'll see them several times," he said. "It's a slow, gentle process."

The Differential Diagnosis: Dr. Right's Main Tool in Finding the Cause of Your Hair Loss

Physicians rely on what is known as a differential diagnosis for finding the possible cause of hair loss and other diseases or conditions. What this means is that they will assess a series of observations, tests, and medical histories, and, like good detectives, they will piece the evidence together to try to get to the bottom of your hair loss. It's not an easy process, and not always definitive.

On your first visit to a dermatologist, "expect a thorough history of past and present medical issues, medications, family history, psychosocial history, as well as a thorough inspection of the scalp, skin, and nails," said

Andrea Lynn Cambio, M.D., a board-certified dermatologist and fellow of the American Academy of Dermatology in private practice in New York City. Cambio and the other physicians I interviewed said dermatologists will also perform blood tests, the "hair pull test," and, in some cases, a scalp biopsy.

Hair Pull Tests and Hair Pluck Tests

The hair pull test, which sounds like some sort of grammar-school hazing, is conducted to rule out telogen effluvium. Wendel explains that the hair pull test tells if you have too many hairs in the shedding, or telogen, phase: "[Shedding] should be a relatively low percentage when you test in various parts of the scalp. In people who are excessively shedding, you'll see that the majority of the hairs, or a greater percentage than should be, are actually in a shedding phase," she says. She notes that the causes of excessive shedding can be things that are often easy to diagnose and treat, "and some of them you just kind of sit out and wait for the hair to return. But I've also found that some women have excessive shedding at the beginning stages of their genetic hair loss, so sometimes it can be deceiving. You get a false sense of confidence that it's going to resolve, when, in fact, it won't."

Nonetheless, Wendel emphasizes the importance of this test, because when it does show a higher-than-normal amount of shedding, it is usually pointing to a temporary cause of hair loss, rather than a permanent cause.

The hair pluck test takes out a bit more hair than the hair pull test, but its goal again is to assess the ratio of telogen hairs to anagen hairs. People with TE may have as much as 50 percent of their hair in the telogen phase, compared to a normal shedding of 10 to 15 percent of hairs on the scalp.

Scalp Biopsy

A scalp biopsy is, as its name implies, the removal of small portions of the scalp, which are then analyzed. Scalp biopsies are not done routinely but may be used to distinguish between chronic telogen effluvium and early stage FPHL, or for the diagnosis of cicatricial alopecia or other scalp conditions.

Blood Tests

Among the blood tests that may be performed are those assessing iron levels, thyroid function, and hormone levels and possibly a test for lupus. In assessing hormone levels, physicians are looking for increased androgen production. (See box on page 54 for a summary of tests).

Testing for Thyroid Disease

Many of the women who wrote to me were concerned that an undiagnosed thyroid disease must be implicated in their hair loss. I asked Cobin about this.

She told me that about 6 percent of the adult population suffers from hypothyroidism and about 2 percent of adults suffer from hyperthyroidism. "As women age, that figure increases. So if you get to be a seventy-year-old woman, odds are about one in ten to fourteen [that you will have thyroid disease]. It's certainly a very common disease, but it doesn't mean everyone has it."

"The part I'm always struck with is that the general, run-of-the-mill doctor doesn't know to look for it. There's a very easy test called TSH [thyroid stimulating hormone]. TSH is cheap, one tube of blood, and even commercial labs run a good TSH, and that's really the most sensitive way to pick up either an under- or an over-active thyroid gland," she explains.

Testing summary

Your physician will use your medical history and pattern of hair loss as the basis for his or her decision about which tests to run. Your physician may request lab tests looking at: FSH (follicle stimulating hormone); LH (leutinizing hormone); thyroid tests including T3, T4, TSH, and thyroid antibody; progesterone and prolactin levels; androgen level assessment (testosterone; DHEA-S); and blood tests. If Lupus is suspected, a special test for the disease will also be run and in some cases, testing for syphilis, a sexually transmitted disease that often causes hair loss, will also be ordered.

She says there's a misconception that seems to crop up periodically on grocery store magazine racks that thyroid can be a hidden and difficult-to-treat disease. "That's a little bit fallacious," she said. "There's some really hokey things out there, like a thermometer under the armpit or measuring thyroid hormone in the urine, that are really not very accurate and really don't give information above and beyond what a good TSH level will give you. Many self-help books are so outside of the mainstream that they're a little misleading."

Cobin explained, however, that sometimes autoimmunity and autoimmune causes can be associated with, but not necessarily caused by, autoimmune thyroid disease, "where we're able to measure, in the blood, anti-thyroid antibodies." She noted that the presence of these antibodies is a good tip-off that something autoimmune-related may be going on, "but that doesn't necessarily mean there is too much or too little thyroid hormone, which can be a cause of hair loss. If there are antibodies present but the thyroid level is normal, there's not a whole lot you can do in manipulating the hormone levels to help for hair loss."

Questions to Consider

The following are questions you should be prepared to answer during your first dermatologist appointment.

- Have you been under any stress lately? Have you experienced job changes, death in the family, or illness, for example?
- Have you recently been pregnant?
- Were you recently ill or hospitalized?
- Did you undergo any recent weight loss due to severe dieting?
- Have you ever been diagnosed with anorexia nervosa or bulimia or any other eating disorder?
- What medications are you taking and why? (Bring them with you, or write down what they are and the dosages.)
- Have you recently started, stopped, or changed your method of oral contraception?
- Do you take hormone replacement therapy (HRT)?
- What vitamins, herbs, and/or homeopathic treatments are you taking? (Bring them with you, or write down what they are, the dosages, and how often you take them.)

But as part of the differential diagnosis, Cobin said, these thyroid antibodies, along with TSH, should be checked and watched. It is possible that with the presence of thyroid antibodies, there may be an underlying autoimmune tendency. Also, since thyroid disease tends to crop up as we age, keeping a close check on your thyroid is not a bad idea.

6

Treatment Talk

Each type of hair loss and various conditions that cause hair loss have some medical treatment options, which this and the following sections will cover. The options outlined below are for you to use as a guide in discussing treatment options with your physician—he or she may have other solutions to offer you as well.

Anagen effluvium, or hair loss resulting from chemotherapy, is an added insult to injury. Studies have shown that for some women, it is the most difficult part of dealing with cancer. Others see anagen effluvium as symbolic of the battle they are fighting against their cancer. Radiation therapy, if it is at or near the head area, can also cause hair loss.

Janet, forty-one, a medical writing colleague, had to cope with hair loss resulting from treatment for her breast cancer. "I guess I thought of the hair loss as part of the package, and a passage I would have to go through," she told me. Janet says she could have chosen a chemotherapy treatment other than Adriamycin that would have had less of an effect on her hair, but she opted not to. "When the oncologist was explaining the choices to my husband and me, I remember saying that I care about my hair, but I would never let that stand in the way of choosing a more effective treatment. I would never forgive myself if my cancer came back and I had chosen a lighter treatment in order to keep my hair," she says. "I wrote an essay about losing my hair, and besides the physical change, the hair was a very visible expression of the destruction going on in my body as the drugs did their deed on any remaining cancer cells."

Janet's husband was also incredibly supportive, which helped her deal with the hair loss. "After my fourth and final chemo, I finally dug out a hand mirror and looked at the back of my head. It actually had a lovely shape. When I told my husband, he said, 'See? I've been telling you all along you look beautiful.'"

If you are facing a battle with cancer, there are some steps you can take to help cope with your hair loss. Keep in mind that the hair loss from cancer treatment is temporary. This may be especially difficult for women who are already dealing with genetic hair loss, but remember that you are fighting a deadly disease, and hair loss may be a consequence, albeit a temporary one.

According to the National Cancer Institute (NCI), not all drugs given to fight cancer cause hair loss, just as Janet's oncologist explained. Your doctor will be able to tell you if the chemotherapy required for your cancer might result in hair loss and whether there are alternative, and equally effective, treatments you can use.

There has been some research on ways to possibly prevent hair loss during chemotherapy treatment, but according to the Mayo Clinic, none has been proven absolutely effective.

Cryotherapy, or scalp hypothermia, in which ice packs or similar devices are placed on your head to slow blood flow to your scalp, have been investigated. "In general, scalp hypothermia works somewhat in 50 percent to 80 percent of people going through chemotherapy who try it. However, the procedure also causes a small risk of cancer recurring in your scalp, as this area doesn't receive the same dose of chemotherapy as the rest of your body," the Mayo Clinic explains on its Web site.

Topical minoxidil (Rogaine) has also been suggested as a way of possibly preventing hair loss from chemotherapy, if applied before and during treatment, but it hasn't been shown to be particularly effective. Some research shows that it may, however, help speed regrowth. A small study cited on the Mayo Clinic's Web site showed that in women who used minoxidil twice daily during their chemotherapy treatment for four months, it took longer for all their hair to fall out compared to women who didn't use it, and the minoxidil users saw hair regrowth about six weeks earlier than the nonusers.

During the course of your treatment, your hair may become thinner or fall out entirely, and the hair loss may occur on all parts of the body. After treatment, the hair will resume its growing cycle, and for some people, hair growth may resume even while still undergoing chemotherapy.

With chemotherapy, the hair loss may not happen right away but can occur several weeks after the first treatment or a few treatments, the NCI says. Some people may experience scalp sensitivity, and the hair may fall out gradually or it may fall out in clumps. The remaining hair may become dull and dry.

Both the NCI and the American Cancer Society advise the following for taking care of your scalp and hair during chemotherapy:

- Use a mild shampoo.
- Use a soft hairbrush.
- Use low heat when drying your hair.
- Don't use brush rollers to set your hair.

- Don't dye your hair or get a permanent.
- Have your hair cut short. A shorter style will make your hair look thicker and fuller. It also will make hair loss easier to manage if it occurs.
- Use a sunscreen, sunblock, hat, scarf, or wig to protect your scalp from the sun.
- Use a satin pillowcase.

Interestingly, after chemotherapy, your hair may grow back in a different texture or color.

Several years ago, I underwent a double breast biopsy, and all signs were pointing toward cancer in at least one breast, if not both. After the initial shock, I seized on an idea. Instead of worrying that chemo might result in my being completely bald for a while, I looked at it as my second chance for hair. I thought that maybe if it all fell out, a new and better head of hair would come in—kind of like bionic hair.

Fortunately, I didn't have to find out.

Janet, however, was not so lucky, and she found various ways to cope as she looked at the bigger picture of her cancer. "I did cry a little at losing my hair," she says. "But I think it was also because it was a symptom of everything I was going through. And I knew, unlike someone with a different (hair) disorder, that it would grow back."

The NCI suggests that if you are considering buying a wig or hairpiece while going through hair loss resulting from chemotherapy, to do so before you lose all your hair so you can get something to match your natural hair color. Of course, you might want to use this time as an opportunity to "try on" a new color as well!

Janet opted for hats and scarves given to her by several friends, including "a great cotton skullcap that I wore a lot . . . In a way, my lack of hair provided a way for some friends to be extra kind to me and lift my spirits while being practical, too."

Hair Loss Myth #4

Hair loss is an evolutionary trait.

Some people have heard that humans lost body hair on their evolutionary path in order to keep cool, so they question if, perhaps, the loss of head hair might serve a similar purpose. Not likely. Scientists don't know why some people lose scalp hair. Furthermore, losing it doesn't appear to point to any of the survival benefits that would qualify as adaptation, which is when nature chooses some traits over others because they aid in the species' survival. Moreover, there is no proof that hair loss is increasing. The hair on your head is mildly beneficial in that it protects the scalp from the elements and provides the skull with padding. Nonetheless, its loss doesn't pose a serious threat.
—*Anita Bhorjee*

Telogen Effluvium

While acute telogen effluvium is usually self-correcting—if you eliminate the triggering event your hair will eventually regrow—chronic telogen effluvium can be difficult to cope with because it is not straightforward. Chronic telogen effluvium (CTE) is generally seen in women between thirty and sixty years old who have a full head of hair before the shedding. "The onset is usually abrupt, with or without a recognizable initiating factor," writes Jerry Shapiro, M.D., in *Hair Loss: Principles of Diagnosis and Management of Alopecia*. In the early stages, he writes, the shedding is usually severe, with the hair "coming out by handfuls." He says the condition does appear to be self-limiting.

The amount of hair shed is more than is seen in female pattern hair loss, but the miniaturization of hairs seen in the genetic disorder is not a feature of chronic telogen effluvium. However, he does explain that the two conditions may coexist.

Shapiro is a clinical professor and director of the Hair Research and Treatment Centre in the Division of Dermatology at the University of British Columbia. At the Centre, CTE is diagnosed by scalp biopsy, and an underlying cause for normal TE is ruled out.

Interestingly, he writes that he prescribes iron plus 5 percent minoxidil twice daily for patients with CTE. "We feel that it is likely that topping up ferritin levels will maximize the hair growth potential of topical minoxidil in those menstruating women with low ferritins," Shapiro says. "However, further studies with double-blinded placebo controls analyzing the single and combinational benefits of supplemental iron and topical minoxidil solution for CTE are needed." So again, you can see the possible importance of serum ferritin in connection with hair loss.

While Shapiro notes chronic telogen effluvium is usually reversible, it can trigger female pattern hair loss, and hair may not return to the same density as it was before the condition started.

Wilma, forty-one, suffered with hair loss for eight years and had originally been diagnosed with female pattern hair loss, but finally found a doctor who realized she was suffering from chronic telogen effluvium. She found that using 5 percent topical minoxidil slowed down the shedding. "My hair is thinner than it was before all this began, but I can see now that I am not going bald. I've gotten on with my life; it doesn't revolve around the hair issue anymore," she told me. "I use Rogaine twice a day but still tend to go through cycles of increased hair loss, but then it goes back to normal."

Wilma's experience indicates the importance of finding proper help, and this point cannot be emphasized enough. She says she didn't believe the diagnosis of female pattern hair loss because "baldness does not run in my family, in men or in women, so genetically, the odds were against me having androgenetic alopecia." Moreover, she said, her hair loss did not progress over time but began with an enormous amount of shedding.

Rhani has found that her chronic telogen effluvium is helped by spironolactone. (More information will be provided about this treatment later in this chapter.)

Alopecia Areata

While there is no FDA-approved treatment for alopecia areata (AA), there are many treatments approved for other conditions that are commonly used for it as well. Because alopecia areata will often go into remission spontaneously, sometimes stopping as suddenly as it began, some people will opt to live with the appearance and disappearance of the bald patches.

However, alopecia areata can be devastating psychologically. Several of the women who wrote to me were suffering from the condition and did not find the treatments they were given helpful; some were dealing with severe depression, and some considered or attempted suicide.

The following medical treatments, outlined by the National Institute of Arthritis and Musculoskeletal and Skin Diseases (NIAMS) have been used for the treatment of AA. While they may help hair regrow, they are not a cure, and there is no guarantee that new bald patches won't reappear.

Corticosteroids

These anti-inflammatory drugs are similar to the hormone cortisol, which the body produces naturally. They work by suppressing the immune system and are used to treat a variety of autoimmune diseases, including alopecia areata, according to NIAMS.

Corticosteroids such as Kenalog can be given through injections into the balding areas, orally (also called systemic therapy), or as a topical ointment or cream. If the injections are successful, hair growth can be seen in about one to two months. They are painful, however, and are not recommended for children.

And while oral corticosteroid therapy is considered a mainstay in treatment for many autoimmune diseases, according to NIAMS it is considered a risky treatment for AA, with many physicians only prescribing corticosteroid use for a very short term. Side effects include hypertension, cataracts, high blood sugar, bone problems, and loss of muscle mass.

Topical corticosteroid treatment is often used for children, as it is not as difficult to deal with as the injections. However, this treatment is less effective than injected corticosteroids and works best when combined with other treatments such as minoxidil or anthralin.

Minoxidil 5 Percent

Topical minoxidil 5 percent, applied twice daily, is often used to help promote hair regrowth in patients with AA. Hair will regrow at about twelve weeks, if it is working.

Anthralin (Psoriatec)

This topical therapy is a treatment for psoriasis that is also used for AA. It is applied for twenty to sixty minutes, but unlike other therapies for this type of hair loss, it is not left on the skin to cause irritation. Hair growth is usually seen in eight to twelve weeks if it is working. Often anthralin is combined with other treatments such as minoxidil or corticosteroids.

Sulfasalazine

This is another drug often used as a treatment for psoriasis. This sulfa drug acts on the immune system and is sometimes used to treat severe cases of the disease. According to questions and answers on the National Alopecia Areata Foundation Web site compiled from a 2002 conference, this treatment has been shown to be effective in some people, but because one study touting its efficacy was retrospective, it is unclear if those who seemingly responded to the drug would have seen their AA resolve without treatment. It has been used as a treatment for long-term colon disease and is relatively safe. The only contraindication to its use is if you have allergies to sulfa or eggs.

Topical Sensitizers

When topical sensitizers, also called topical immunotherapy, are applied to the scalp, they cause an allergic reaction marked by itching and scaling, according to NIAMS. New hair growth, if the treatment is effective, occurs in three to twelve months. Squaric acid dibutyl ester (SADBE) and diphenylcyclopropenone (DPCP) are two topical sensitizers often used for AA; however, their s clinicafety and the consistency of their formulation are currently under review.

An article reviewing treatments from the University of British Columbia Hair Clinic where Jerry Shapiro, M.D., is director, cites a study where researchers treated 139 patients with DPCP for one year, which showed that 50.4 percent of the patients had either total regrowth or a "satisfactory" response with only a few remaining bald patches. Gradual discontinuance of the treatment did not appear to affect the regrowth. Success rate, the article noted, is influenced by the extent and duration of hair loss, with less success in patients with alopecia totalis or universalis and a long duration of the disease before therapy.

The article notes that at the clinic they use DPCP in patients with more than 50 percent hair loss from AA and recommends that it should only be used under the supervision of dermatologists. This is probably a good suggestion for all these therapies.

Duvic told me that topical sensitizers result in a contact dermatitis (a rash) that generates a T-cell response. The immune system reacts to the rash—which acts as a decoy—instead of attacking the hair follicle. For some people, this will result in hair regrowth. It's not an easy treatment, but it's certainly worth pursuing if nothing else has worked.

Oral Cyclosporine

Cyclosporine is used as a treatment to keep people from rejecting transplanted organs and as an immunosuppressant in psoriasis and other autoimmune skin conditions. Because of the side effects of this treatment, which include an increased risk of serious infection and a possibility of developing a type of skin cancer, physicians often feel the risks outweigh the possible benefits of the drug's use in treating AA. And while it may help regrow hair, it is not a cure.

Photochemotherapy (PUVA)

A light-sensitive drug called psoralen, given either orally or as a topical cream and then exposed to ultraviolet light, has been shown in clinical studies to cause "cosmetically acceptable hair re-growth" in about 55 percent of people undergoing the therapy. Such a success rate sounds great, but the relapse rate is high, it requires treatment two to three times a week at a clinic, and it carries the risk of developing skin cancer.

Experimental Treatments for AA

Cindy was beside herself on how to deal with her AA until she found a doctor using an experimental treatment at UCLA—a topical immunotherapy treatment called dinitrochlorobenzene (DNCB). The treatment works like the topical sensitizers discussed above. Cindy says that after three painful years of other treatments failing, she now has hair on 90 percent of her head with the use of DNCB. I relay Cindy's story to let you know that although she found a UCLA School of Medicine dermatologist who is using this ointment in his practice and presumably having good luck with it, I am not sure it is widely available. And like most treatments, it may not work or be tolerable for everyone. I called the doctor's office several times to learn more about this, but I could not get an interview with him for this book.

Nonetheless, a study published in the *Archives of Dermatology* does suggest that in a small study of eighty patients, the treatment proved effective. The study was well designed in that it was a half-head study, meaning each patient was treated with the ointment on one half of the head, which was then compared to the untreated half, so that if spontaneous remission were occurring, it would temper the results seen with the treatment. The researchers found that 89 percent of the patients in the study either regrew hair exclusively on the treated side of the head, or it grew considerably faster or denser, and the difference was seen in eight weeks. The researchers add, "The initial response, however, could not be maintained in all of these patients. Persistent response was observed in seventy-two patients (80 percent)."

Ongoing Research

Duvic says that at M. D. Anderson's Melanoma and Skin Center they are currently studying a vitamin A analogue that was developed for cutaneous T-cell lymphoma. "Patients with cutaneous T-cell lymphoma often have alopecia areata with malignant or stimulating clonal T-cells for the hair follicles. We noticed that some of the people on this type of vitamin A were growing their hair back, so we have a trial of these topical agents ongoing right now," she says. The trial is currently in Phase II, the second of three stages required to seek FDA approval of a drug.

Enbrel and Raptiva, two drugs used to treat rheumatoid arthritis and psoriasis, are also being tested for their efficacy in alopecia areata.

For more information on alopecia areata, visit www.naaf.org, and, if you suffer from this disease, also sign up for the previously mentioned National Alopecia Areata Registry.

"It's very important to join the registry, because we are collecting information in association with other autoimmune diseases, and everyone who registers goes into the epidemiology study of self-registered patients. And we're inviting patients that have certain subtypes or family histories to come in and have blood samples drawn," Duvic, who heads the registry, says. "We're setting up lymphoblast lines, DNA, and sera that will be provided to researchers, so it will be a tool for further research." At the time this book was written, four thousand people had registered, and blood samples had been collected on three hundred and fifty to four hundred people.

Medical Treatments for Other Types of Hair Loss

Cicatricial Alopecias

These types of hair loss usually progress along an irreversible course, because they destroy the hair follicle. Steroids injected into the lesions or drugs used for malaria are sometimes used to treat the condition.

Trichtotillomania

Because this type of hair loss is considered a psychological disorder, it is usually treated with medications used for the treatment of depression or obsessive-compulsive disorder, such as selective serotonin reuptake inhibitors (SSRIs) like Paxil, Wellbutrin, or Lexapro.

Female Pattern Hair Loss

The biggest problem with female pattern hair loss is that outside of understanding that there is a genetic cause, not much else is known. Moreover, there is not a wealth of research in this area, and what there is, more often than not, yields as many questions as answers.

"We understand the male pattern hair loss much better than women's hair loss, and understand better the role of androgens in that process. To answer the question of what's going on with women is much, much more challenging than in men, because it's just poorly understood. Women's hair loss doesn't follow the same pathways as men's," Haber says. Speaking about FPHL specifically, he says that typically there is an acceleration of hair loss after menopause, but it will also often show up at age eighteen or nineteen.

While there are some conditions, such as PCOS, where there is a direct connection between a woman's hair loss and excess androgens, Dr. Haber and other doctors I

Hair Loss Myth #5

Improving circulation will cure hair loss.

Not true—but this myth has proved the hardest to shake of them all, and it still has proponents in traditional and natural medicine. Advice is given to do headstands, perform scalp massages, or even rub pastes on the scalp made from "stimulating ingredients" such as cayenne pepper to improve blood flow to the scalp. While more outlandish instruments to increase circulation to the scalp, such as applying a spark with an electrode, are things of the distant past, this theory was still being toyed with as recently as a decade ago. In 1992, a Canadian company believed it had a promising approach to hair loss by applying low-powered electrical impulses to the scalp using a helmet-like hood. The failure of this endeavor may have finally put this theory to rest. But don't bet on it.

—*Anita Bhorjee*

interviewed say that clear-cut hormonal associations are rare. "But certainly they have hair loss, and they don't respond to the anti-androgen approaches," Haber says.

Draelos points out that there are more patterns of hair loss in females than in males. "In some women, the hair loss spares the anterior [frontal] hairline and they have thinning on top; some have bitemporal recessions [thinning at the temples]; some just have an overall thinning; while others lose their hair just at the crown."

So while conventional medical treatments aimed at controlling excess androgen can reverse hair loss in men, they may not work at all in many women. But they do work for some.

There is only one product approved by the FDA that is allowed to make claims that it can actually regrow hair in women: topical minoxidil, sold commercially as Rogaine. This book devotes a lot of space to minoxidil, not because it works the best, but because it is the one product we know the most about. And no matter what type of hair loss you have, it will likely be the one product recommended for you to try.

Nonetheless, despite the attention I devote to it, as I said at the outset, I don't feel it is right to tout a particular treatment or say that a specific regimen will reverse your hair loss. That's not what this book is about. I am not endorsing topical minoxidil or any other product or regimen as a preferred treatment for hair loss.

My focus is to compile most of what we know and, I hope, give a perspective on some of the more established or well-known treatments out there that you may encounter in your quest to find the best treatment for your situation. I've included information on side effects. For each woman who may benefit from a particular treatment, there will also be many who won't see much, if any, improvement at all.

CAUTION: Before using any of the products listed below, read the labels for contraindications (reasons not to take it), and discuss its use with your physician if you are unsure about any of the precautions. You should always be aware of possible side effects; keep in mind that labels must reflect any problem that arose during the testing of a product even if it only occurred in one person. Take particular care if you are pregnant or planning to become pregnant, as some of the treatments included here have mostly been tested in men.

Topical Treatments for FPHL

Topical treatments are those that are applied directly to the scalp. Their advantage, for the most part, is that they are safe; their drawback is that they can be difficult to apply, messy, or make hair styling difficult.

Topical Minoxidil (Rogaine)

Topical minoxidil solution, the generic name for Rogaine, is the best-known, and the only FDA-approved, treatment for hair loss in women. It's one you may already be using, have tried, or be thinking about trying.

It is not known exactly how minoxidil works, but what is known is how it affects the hair follicles. The treatment appears to increase the anagen phase of hair growth and also enlarges the hair follicles, resulting in vellus (peach-fuzz hairs) becoming enlarged and converting to terminal hair. Shedding is also decreased.

Clinical data: A forty-eight-week, double-blind, placebo-controlled, randomized trial showed that women using minoxidil 2 percent had a 29 percent increase in hair counts and a 42 percent increase in hair weight over a thirty-two-week period.

Clinical data from studies conducted by Pharmacia (now Pfizer), the manufacturer of Rogaine, reported that in women with mild to moderate hair loss, 19 percent had moderate regrowth and 40 percent had minimal regrowth after using the product for eight months, compared to 7 percent moderate regrowth and 33 percent minimal regrowth for those women given a placebo. Most of the women participating in the studies were Caucasian, ages eighteen to forty-five.

Most common side effects: scalp irritation and increased shedding with initial use, which usually abate on their own. (See Appendix C for ways to deal with this.) Hypertrichosis, or excessive hair growth, usually on the face, affects 3 to 5 percent of women using the 2 percent solution, and more than 5 percent of those using the 5 percent dosage. Hypertrichosis will usually disappear after a year even if you continue to use minoxidil. If you stop the treatment, it will abate within one to six months.

Other side effects: While not common, other possible side effects that could be associated with the use of topical minoxidil include chest pain, rapid heartbeat, faintness, dizziness, and swelling of the hands or feet. The product should be stopped if you experience any of these.

As these data show, it is obvious that topical minoxidil is not the magic bullet for stopping women's hair loss.

Ketoconazole (Nizoral Shampoo)

A study in 1998 compared using shampoo containing ketoconazole two to four times a week with using topical minoxidil. The researchers found that the treatment was comparable, with a positive effect on hair density and size, as well as on the proportion of hairs in the anagen phase.

The study concluded that regular use of shampoo containing 2 percent ketoconazole may help improve genetic hair loss. Unfortunately, the 1998 trial was small in size, and the authors recommended that a larger controlled study was necessary to confirm the results. So far, this larger trial has not been conducted.

Nonetheless, since ketoconazole is available commercially as a shampoo called Nizoral and is available on pharmacy and grocery shelves without a prescription, it is certainly worth a try, as it appears from this small study and anecdotal reports that its efficacy is possibly on par with minoxidil.

Ketoconazole can also help with the itch and inflammation related to hair loss. Wendel told me that biopsies have confirmed an inflammatory response to hair loss in some people. "I do recommend ketoconazole to my patients for use once or twice a week, depending on how often they shampoo," she says. "It has been shown to decrease the inflammatory response [associated with hair loss] and probably has limited benefit in terms of its testosterone inhibition as well, but it really needs to stay on the scalp for a good three to five minutes before washing it out."

Ketoconazole is also a well-documented treatment for dandruff and seborrhea, which may also be contributing to your hair loss.

Tricomin Products

I debated whether to put these products here or in the section on hair care products. Because these treatments, which include a shampoo, conditioner, and scalp spray, have a bit of science behind their development, I decided to list them here.

Tricomin products are made by the Procyte Corporation, which also makes GraftCyte, a topical peptide copper acetate that is used after hair transplantation to expedite healing of the grafts. Tricomin products contain this copper-binding peptide, which the company is promoting as a possible help with hair loss. It has been available commercially since 1996. While some users have reported that the products have helped with hair growth, most have said the existing hair appears strengthened.

Wendel says she recommends Tricomin products to her patients, as they are reasonably priced and their statements for efficacy are backed by some clinical research. The Tricomin spray, which has a higher concentration of the active ingredient, is healing to the scalp for women who may be experiencing irritation with use of topical minoxidil, she said.

Systemic Treatments

Systemic treatments are drugs or other treatments taken by mouth that may positively affect your hair, but which also may affect your whole body. And because they are usually treatments for other conditions, their use may be associated with adverse side effects. These treatments should be used with caution and only under a physician's guidance, especially if you have other underlying medical problems or are pregnant or may become pregnant. Many of the products require you to be on oral contraceptives (birth-control pills) if you are using them and could become pregnant, as they may harm a fetus.

Spironolactone (Aldactone)

Spironolactone, a treatment originally developed as a treatment for hypertension (high blood pressure), has been getting a lot of press as a possible treatment for female pattern hair loss, and nearly everyone who wrote to me was either trying it or wanting to try it.

The FDA has not approved spironolactone, which is sold by prescription as Aldactone, for any dermatologic conditions, including hair loss. While this is a very popular treatment, Haber told me there is very little evidence that it works. "There are no studies that are 'wow' for the drug," he says.

In his article on pharmacologic treatments for hair loss, Haber writes, "Its antiandrogen properties are weak, and high dosages and long-term therapy are necessary to see any clinical benefit."

Haber says he is most likely to recommend the treatment if a woman is hyperandrogenic with PCOS or hirsutism. "But I'll also use it in a woman who is eager to try anything and is not a candidate for Propecia, who has tried Rogaine and it's not working, and they want to try something else," Haber says. (See below for information on Propecia.) He assesses the lab work at three, six, nine, and twelve months.

Some of the side effects associated with the drug may self-correct within two to three months of starting therapy, and if they do not, decreasing the dosage to 50 to 75 milligrams a day may help. However, since the dosage that seems to be most effective for hair loss is 200 milligrams per day, cutting back the dosage would likely undermine its efficacy.

Possible side effects: Spironolactone crosses the placenta barrier and can cause feminization of a male fetus. Oral contraceptives must be taken if you are considering using this drug and could become pregnant. Other side effects include menstrual irregularities, hyperkalemia (high potassium levels), and electrolyte abnormalities.

NOTE: Spironolactone should not be used by women with a genetic risk for breast cancer.

Possible drug interactions: Spironolactone should not be used if you are taking other potassium-sparing diuretics or if you are taking salicylates, ACE inhibitors, digitalis, or digoxin. Consult your doctor about its use if you are breast-feeding, as spironolactone has been detected in breast milk.

Cimetidine (Tagamet)

Cimetidine, sold commercially as Tagamet, is a well-established treatment for duodenal ulcers and other conditions. It is also an antiandrogen, which is what put it on the radar for use in hair loss. It is used off-label (not for what the medication was originally intended) for the treatment of genetic baldness and hirsutism in women. No clinical data, however, have shown its efficacy. The recommended dosage for hair loss is 800 to 1600 milligrams a day, given orally in 300 milligram doses five times daily.

Finasteride (Propecia)

Finasteride, which is sold under the brand name Propecia, is a type II 5-alpha reductase inhibitor, which is the most common isotope found in the hair follicle. The drug is administered orally in a 1-milligram daily dose. While highly effective as a hair loss treatment for men, it is only indicated for use in a small subset of women, and because it can cause abnormalities in a developing fetus, it should not be used by women of childbearing age who could become pregnant.

"I do use it in a small subset of female patients, but I can't agree to an objective clarity that it's working, but they don't seem to be getting any worse," Haber says. "I haven't put a new woman on [Propecia] in several years, but it's something for the appropriately screened woman. I won't put a woman on it who has any possibility of getting pregnant, but I will use it in postmenopausal/sterile women. But I'm honest with these women and tell them there is no scientific evidence that it works whatsoever and that they might be wasting their money," he adds. He notes that the lack of study of finasteride's effect in women is likely due to its side effects.

Clinical studies: One yearlong, prospective, placebo-controlled, double-blind study of the drug's use in postmenopausal women with FPHL did not show either a slowing of hair loss or promotion of hair growth. Another, more recent study did show that four women with hirsutism with elevated testosterone and other lab abnormalities did respond to the drug, which suggests it may be beneficial for a small subset of women with FPHL.

Cyproterone Acetate (Cyprostat)

Cyproterone acetate, sold commercially as Cyprostat, is a drug used as a treatment for prostate cancer and benign prostatic hypertrophy (enlarged prostate). It is used off-label in FPHL and hirsutism. The dosage for FPHL is 100 milligrams a day taken on days five to fourteen of the menstrual cycle. It can be used in combination with the oral contraceptive Demulan and seems to stabilize hair loss, meaning it won't necessarily regrow hair but may keep shedding from getting any worse.

This drug is most effective for women who have clinical evidence of hyperandrogenism such as acne, hirsutism, menstrual irregularities, and a high body mass index.

Possible side effects: menstrual irregularities, weight gain, breast tenderness, and feminization of a male fetus. If women of childbearing age who could become pregnant are going to try this, they must use an oral contraceptive to prevent pregnancy. In a recent study of women taking this drug for FPHL, some reported shortness of breath.

NOTE: Cyproterone acetate is not available in the United States, but it is available in Canada and Europe.

Flutamide (Eulexin)

Flutamide, sold under the brand name Eulexin, is an antiandrogen drug used for the treatment of prostate cancer.

A study comparing the use of flutamide with cyproterone acetate and finasteride in forty-eight women with hyperandrogenism who were treated daily for one year, found that flutamide had a significant impact on hair loss over the other two treatments.

Possible side effects: significant incidence of liver toxicity, including liver failure. It may harm the fetus if used by a women who is pregnant.

Oral Contraceptives

The area of hormones, as I stated before, is fraught with controversy. Starting, stopping, or changing doses of oral contraceptives can either help or hurt hair loss, or have no effect. While it seems there should be a direct relationship between estrogen and hair loss, it's weak at best.

If you are using the drugs for contraception and suffering from FPHL, ask your physician for the type that will least affect your hair. Birth-control pills containing the least amount of androgenic progestin, such as norgestimate (Ortho Cyclen, Ortho Tri-Cyclen), norethindrone (Ovcon 35), desogestrel (Mircette, Desogen), and ethynodiol diacetate (Demulen, Zovia), appear to least affect hair loss.

Yasmin, which contains estradiol and drospirenone, an analogue of spironolactone, may even help hair loss for some women. Each pill contains the equivalent of 25 milligrams of spironolactone. The drug is often prescribed for women with FPHL who are also seeking birth control. However, there have not been any studies showing specifically that the pill prevents hair loss or promotes hair regrowth.

Because birth-control pills can mimic the hormonal environment of pregnancy, they can cause temporary hair loss when they are started or stopped, says Nanette Santoro, M.D., professor and director of the division of reproductive endocrinology at Albert Einstein College of Medicine, New York. "Women trying to avoid hair loss from contraceptive pills might want to start with the lowest progestin dose available, but there's no clear guidance on this. It's best to relate this concern to one's physician and make an informed choice," she says.

Wendel recommends that young women losing their hair take birth-control pills and says that Yasmin is her first choice for these patients.

Possible side effects: breast tenderness, nausea, headache, mood swings, painful menstruation, bleeding between periods, and depression. These side effects are common to most oral contraceptives.

Hormone Replacement Therapy (HRT)

As you enter menopause, you may begin to notice hair loss for the first time, or if you have already been coping with female pattern hair loss, it may seem to worsen.

Is it the loss of estrogen at this time of life that causes hair loss, and will hormone replacement therapy help the condition, along with alleviating hot flashes, night sweats, and vaginal dryness? Not an easy question to answer, as I found out when I posed it to the medical experts I interviewed.

"Certainly more women begin to lose their hair after menopause," Haber says. "Is [menopause] triggering a genetic susceptibility, or is it . . . age-related, non-genetic, slow organ failure?" he says, referring to the fact that as we get older some bodily functions begin to slow down, and hair, unfortunately, can be susceptible to that process. How estrogen loss factors into that rubric, and whether HRT can help hair loss, is another thorny question.

Haber and most of the medical experts I spoke with do not see HRT as a reliable treatment for hair loss. Some women swear it helps; others find, just as with oral contraception, that it either does not help at all or worsens the condition.

The risks of using HRT need to be weighed against the possible beneficial effect it may have on your hair.

"The issue of hormone replacement therapy in post-menopausal women is a very hot topic right now. If a woman has a strong family history of breast, uterine, or ovarian cancer, or a strong family history of heart disease, then hormones are definitely contraindicated. This rules out a lot of women, because the major cause of death in women is heart disease, followed by cancer," says Wendel.

The Women's Health Initiative, a fifteen-year program launched in 1991 consisting of clinical trials and observational study of more than 161,000 postmenopausal women, looked at hormone therapy as well as other treatments to determine the most common causes of death, disability, and poor quality of life. The researchers concluded that estrogen plus progestin therapy increased a woman's risk of heart attack, stroke, and blood clots. In the portion of the study that looked at estrogen alone, there was an increased risk of stroke and blood clots. (Estrogen-only therapy should not be used by postmenopausal women with an intact uterus.)

While some benefits were found with the use of HRT, the researchers concluded that its risk outweighs its benefit other than for use by women with severe symptoms of menopause, such as hot flashes, night sweats, and vaginal dryness. The FDA now recommends that HRT should be used only at the lowest effective dose and for the shortest amount of time for control of menopausal symptoms.

"I personally wouldn't recommend HRT now until more research is done," Wendel says. "I have seen many women who are still on HRT despite the findings of the Women's Health Initiative, and they have no intention of coming off them for fear of more hair loss. I inform them of their risks, and they understand them but are so upset with their hair loss that their primary doctors or gynecologists have agreed to keep them on the therapy for now, with the hope of stopping it in the near future."

Cobin concurs. She told me it's a tough call for advising women with hair loss on HRT use. "It's not usually the case that severe cases of alopecia are from estrogen deficiency per se," she says. "If that were the case, all menopausal women would be losing their hair, and we know that's not true."

Nonetheless, if you do not have a high risk for breast cancer or cardiovascular disease and do find that HRT seems to be helping your hair loss, discuss your dosage and the duration of your treatment with your gynecologist and dermatologist. Be sure to maintain your cardio-vascular health through diet and exercise, and get regular gynecologic checkups, including yearly mammograms.

Other Treatments

Saw Palmetto (*Serenoa Repens*)

Saw palmetto is a well-known and well-studied herb for the treatment of benign prostatic hypertrophy (enlarged prostate) in men. It's known to inhibit 5 alpha-reductase levels by 32 percent without affecting testosterone levels, and it appears to have a partial antagonistic effect on testosterone receptors. While it is reported as being relatively safe, causing gastrointestinal distress in some, this herb has been studied mostly in men. Women should note any unusual side effects, especially menstrual irregularities. One woman who wrote to me told me that saw palmetto caused her to have extremely difficult menses. Discuss use of saw palmetto with your gynecologist, especially if you are pregnant or are planning to become pregnant.

Possible side effects: gastrointestinal upset. Also, women using saw palmetto should watch for menstrual problems and probably not use it if they are pregnant or trying to become pregnant.

The Pregnancy Dilemma

Deciding what treatments to try for hair loss is particularly difficult for young women of childbearing age who hope to have children one day. While early treatment is suggested for treating hair loss, all of the treatments carry possible concerns for pregnant women. Even topical minoxidil, which is considered the safest treatment, shouldn't be taken without consulting your physician if you are pregnant.

Rhani voices this concern: "I am at the age where I want to settle down and have children very much, but going off the spironolactone will definitely have an awful effect on my hair and face." She fears that if it takes six months to a year to get pregnant, her skin and hair will be a mess by the time she gives birth and finishes breast-feeding. "It seems awful that the one thing I want so much—motherhood—is the same thing I am so afraid of. Not to mention that I wonder if I could have done myself any harm through saw palmetto or spironolactone."

I think that of all the women writing to me, young women like Rhani break my heart the most. They are at an age when their world is opening before them as they zero in on careers, relationships, and the possibility of motherhood. Why should these women have to think about sacrificing their hair for the possibility of having children? Some are so psychologically devastated by their hair loss that they cannot even fathom the choice because they are too depressed to consider the consequences.

Someone not going through hair loss might see such choices as a no-brainer—of course you opt for the health; you opt for the child. Haber told me about a patient who had severe psoriasis and found a treatment that miraculously cleared it up; for the first time in his life, he had normal skin. The drug had a devastating side effect, however, and he ended up on dialysis to save his kidneys. Once his organ health was restored, he begged to be put back on the drug! Insane? Perhaps, but given what appearance means in today's society, it's completely understandable if you are going through such a dilemma. Women losing their hair can identify with this gentleman.

If you are pregnant or considering getting pregnant, talk about your options for your hair loss with your physicians and have them help you map out a plan to get through it. The one good thing about pregnancy is that for its duration, most of us gain a bit of hair as the shedding stage slows way down.

Of course, the best aspect of pregnancy is the wonderful bundle of joy you will bring into the world. Take all precautions to ensure that he or she thrives in the most healthy pregnancy environment possible!

Surgical Treatment Options

"Hair transplantation is my golden apple," Rhani told me. "The women in my family lose their hair noticeably after giving birth, and if I am ever lucky enough to give birth, I plan to have a hair transplant at that point," she says.

Since medical treatments are not the answer for everyone, is hair transplantation the Holy Grail for treating hair loss in women?

No, but like the other treatments, it may help some women, especially those with FPHL.

Christine, sixty-four, always had fine hair, but when she was pregnant in the 1960s she noticed balding at the crown, and while she asked her doctors about her hair loss and they ran the usual tests, everything came back normal. There were no treatments for hair loss back then, especially in women, so once the obvious causes were eliminated, Christine was left with no answers or possible help for her FPHL.

Several years ago, Christine consulted with a hair restoration surgeon and had a hair transplant of six hundred hairs from the back of her head to the crown. "I used to cry every day before I had the hair transplantation," she writes. "Since then, I am a lot happier and I don't worry about my hair as much. It's still very thin, and I was told by the hair restoration physician that I needed another four hundred grafts, but I just couldn't afford it." Christine says that if she is financially able, she will have another transplant.

Hair transplantation, or hair restoration surgery, wasn't always considered a viable option for women. But the procedure has evolved from the earlier "doll-head" look of the old-fashioned, telltale hair-plug procedure to one that is more refined and aesthetically pleasing.

The latest technology and procedures, as well as the aesthetic sensibilities of the many physicians now performing hair restoration surgery, have transformed it into a viable option for women.

"For many years, traditionally trained hair transplant doctors never considered the procedure in women," says Jeff Epstein, M.D., a hair transplant surgeon in private practice in Boca Raton and Miami, Florida. This is because the earlier technique, even one that first improved on the doll-head look, was more suited to men with areas of complete baldness.

In reality, the hair-plug procedure was skin grafting—a section of bald skin was replaced with a piece of skin that had hairs in it. For men, even this earlier procedure was a win-win situation, as the patch of skin was taken from a place with hair and placed in an area that had no hair. This couldn't be used successfully in women with diffuse thinning or a widening part not completely devoid of hairs, as the placement of the graft would cause trauma to the surrounding hairs.

However, the procedure evolved. Instead of moving sections of skin with hair, hair restoration surgeons now move hair follicles. There are two major techniques now used: mini-micrografting and follicular unit transplantation, with the latter considered the procedure that produces the most natural-looking and aesthetically pleasing result. "The big advantage for a woman is that the recipient site can be smaller, with less trauma to existing [surrounding] hairs," Epstein says.

To learn more about the procedures, visit www.foundhair.com, www.bosley.com, www.newhair.com, or www.HairLossTalk.com. For the purposes of this book, I want to focus most on what you can expect from this option.

Assessing Candidates for Hair Restoration Surgery

As stated at the beginning of this chapter, hair restoration surgery is not a viable option for all women. This is because in order to successfully transplant hair to your bald or thinning areas, called the recipient sites, you must have a place on your head that has enough hair to spare. This area is called the donor site, and it is usually at the back of the head.

Your hair restoration surgeon will assess your scalp to make sure you have a viable donor site. If you have diffuse thinning over your entire head, you are likely not a good candidate for a hair transplant for two reasons—one, there is not a good donor site, and two, with overall diffuse thinning it means all the hairs on your head are programmed to shed.

The reason hair transplantation works in some people is that the hairs taken from the donor site are not programmed to fall out as they are in the balding areas. This is why most bald men have a fairly thick fringe surrounding their central balding area. When the hair from the donor site is put into the area of hair loss, the donor hairs keep their genetically coded programming.

"It's a horrible thing to hear when you go [for consultation] that you are not an appropriate candidate, but at the same time, you don't want to go through with it if it's not right for you," Ken Washenik, M.D., medical director of Bosley Medical Center, explains. "It's a big event in your life, it's a big expense, and the only reason you're doing it is to gain the benefit."

Additionally, the doctors I interviewed told me any underlying medical condition such as thyroid disease should be stabilized before hair transplantation is undertaken. This is important so the physician has a clear idea of whether the hair is stable enough to undergo the procedure.

Hair transplantation should not be the first choice in treating your hair loss, but if a visit to a hair restoration surgeon is your first doctor's visit in regard to your hair, you will—or should—be put through the same battery of tests a dermatologist would put you through. This, of course, is to ensure that if you have a treatable condition or underlying medical condition, it is taken care of. Then the hair transplant option becomes clearer as to what it can or cannot do for your situation.

High Hopes and a Dose of Reality

Wendel said that about 20 percent of the patients she sees for hair loss choose hair restoration surgery. She noted that women have extremely high expectations of what hair transplantation can do for them and what it cannot do. "The important thing that they need to understand with surgery is that it isn't going to make them have the hair they had when they were twenty-five. It doesn't work that way," she says.

While the surgery will make you look better than you do now, it won't restore your hair to what you had before you began to lose your hair, nor will it transform you into Heather Locklear. All the hair restoration surgeons I spoke with said that patients need to come to terms with this before they agree to surgery. Moreover, if you are seeking consultation for a hair transplant and this reality

is not made clear to you or the procedure is not presented in a realistic light, get another opinion. It is better to
expect a small return from the procedure and be pleas-
antly surprised than to have false expectations and be dis-
appointed.

Once a patient accepts the reality of what hair restoration surgery can and cannot do, the surgeon will paint a
realistic picture, saying: This will look better; this won't
change; will you be happy with that? "And we make that
point over and over again, and the success rate is good,"
Wendel says.

But it gets worse before it gets better.

Because the hair follicle, which is the important part of
the procedure, is transplanted, the hairs moved to the
new location fall out within three weeks of the surgery,
and new hair does not begin growing until around the
third month. In about six to eight months, about 90 percent of the finished results will be noticeable.

There will be scabbing of the incisions right after the
surgery, so you're not going to emerge from the surgical
suite looking like you just stepped out of the salon with
new, flowing locks. This is not a quick fix, and the good
results of the procedure will not be noticeable for some
months. Wendel noted that it takes a whole year and
patience before the full benefits are seen.

Most transplant surgeons advise their patients to continue using topical minoxidil if they are already doing
so. "Use of minoxidil before the transplant procedure
and three months after decreases shedding," Wendel
explained. "And even for people who are opposed to
Rogaine, we really push its use for this peri-operative
phase." And if minoxidil is working for you in keeping
the hair you still have, continuing its use after the transplant is crucial, the physicians advised. GraftCyte may
also be prescribed after the procedure to aid in the healing of the transplanted areas.

"Hair transplantation is a treatment, not a cure," says Epstein. "We're not doing anything to stop the natural progression of hair loss, so the original [nontransplanted] hair will continue to fall out. While transplants are called 'permanent,' I do counsel patients that as you get older, you will have a 10 to 20 percent thinning of the transplants." The usual progression of aging, along with the usual progression of FPHL, will continue to take its toll, with the exception that the transplanted hairs will tend to be more viable longer.

But the artistry of the procedure is how the new hairs are distributed, and your surgeon will discuss this with you. "One of the things that is not done is getting every hair back that you started with. You're taking a smaller number of hairs and redistributing them for maximum coverage and benefit," Washenik explains. "This differs from one person to the next. Someone may really want hair in the front, someone may really want hair in the back, and someone may have developed thinning everywhere, but it's especially noticeable down where they part their hair on one side." He explains that surgeons use a concept called "differential density" to concentrate the hair where it's of most use to the patient.

Should hair restoration surgery be undertaken before, during, or after menopause?

"The time to have a transplant is when (the hair loss) bothers the patient the most," Epstein says. Again, the natural aging process, as well as the effect of FPHL on nontransplanted hairs in the thinning areas, will continue to take its toll. "With the continuation of menopause, they may continue to lose more hair, but they're not going to be worse off if they hadn't done it, as they'll always have the benefit of the transplant," Epstein says.

And remember, if you do have a viable donor site and you can afford the procedure, you can have additional transplants as time goes on.

Hair Restoration Surgery for
African American Women

Hair restoration surgery is also a viable option for African American women with FPHL who are candidates with good donor sites. However, there are some differences in the procedure that you should be aware of, and you should make sure you choose a surgeon who is experienced in working on African American hair.

Since African Americans are sometimes prone to keloid scarring, your surgeon should take a careful history to determine if you are at risk for this sort of scarring. Topical corticosteroids and an antibiotic ointment applied for two weeks after the procedure have been shown to help prevent this scarring.

Choosing a Surgeon

There is no board certification by the American Board of Medical Specialties (ABMS) for hair restoration surgeons. Let me say it again: The ABMS, the "board" in the phrase "board-certified physician," does not have a certification for hair restoration surgeons.

Epstein, for instance, is ABMS-certified in otolaryngology—head and neck surgery. Doctors who are board certified are usually certified under one or more ABMS specialty.

However, Epstein explains, hair specialists have taken it upon themselves to form the American Board of Hair Restoration Surgery (ABHRS), which is a non-ABMS-approved board that serves as a consumer-protection type of organization that "lets the prospective patient know that at least their physician has passed some type of basic competency exam." This certification cannot be advertised without a disclaimer that it is a non-ABMS board.

"I think it makes sense to expect that the doctors who are doing hair transplants be certified in at least one

ABMS board and, in addition, be certified by the American Board of Hair Restoration Surgery, just from a consumer-protection stance," Epstein says. "It is likely that in the next six to ten years the ABHRS will try to achieve equivalency with one of the ABMS boards, such as what the American Board of Facial, Plastic, and Reconstructive Surgery has done, which is a sub-board of the American Board of Otolaryngology."

Along with thoroughly checking out your doctor—which should include an initial consultation, a look at "before and after" pictures of other hair transplant patients, and a thorough assessment of what can or cannot be done for you—make sure to determine the doctor's credentials. If his or her board certification is not clear, don't be afraid to ask.

It is fairly common practice now for hair restoration surgeons, like other doctors, to have Web sites. Check them out, and check out other doctors from around the country in order to compare all the treatment options, as well as their credentials.

Is hair restoration surgery right for you?

- Consult with a physician to rule out any other health conditions causing your hair loss, and have these treated first.
- Do you have a good donor site?
- Are your expectations realistic?
- Discuss with your surgeon exactly what can be done for your particular hair loss.
- Ask to review "before and after" pictures of patients who have undergone the procedure,

paying close attention to women whose "before" pictures most match your particular hair loss.

- Ask to talk to patients who have had the procedure done.
- Remember that photos are taken with diffuse light and hair often looks thicker in photos than in person. Discuss this with your surgeon.
- Consider starting with a small procedure first, perhaps in the frontal area, and then returning for another procedure in a year or so. This will let you see how your expectations match reality, as well as enable you to see how the procedure "takes" for you.
- Can you afford it? Hair restoration procedures are rarely covered by health insurance and, at the time this book was written, typically cost anywhere from $5,000 to $10,000 (the amount can vary depending on the number of grafts).
- Are you willing to undergo the possible post-surgical crusting and shedding, and can you cope with not seeing the positive results of the surgery for nearly a year?
- The good news is that studies have shown that on average, about 80 to 90 percent of the grafted (transplanted) hairs grow in the recipient site. Some surgeons claim even higher success rates, so discuss this with your surgeon.

7

Special Hair Loss Concerns for African American Women

The occurrence and treatment of telogen effluvium, alopecia areata, female pattern hair loss, and other common forms of alopecia are the same for African American women as for their Caucasian counterparts, according to Valerie Callender, M.D., of the Callender Skin and Laser Center in Mitchellville, Maryland. However, Callender and her colleagues, writing in the journal *Dermatologic Therapy*, point out that some forms of hair loss are more common in the black population or are a cause for special concern in light of hairstyling practices. These include female pattern hair loss (treatment concerns), trichorrhexis nodosa, traction alopecia, seborrheic dermatitis, and central centrifugal cicatricial alopecia.

Trichorrhexis nodosa is a type of hair-shaft damage that results from physical or chemical trauma. "Presumably, the decreased tensile strength of chemically treated hair in African Americans, heat exposure, and other drying agents play a role in the development of breakage," Callender writes. "The involved hairs often break a few centimeters from the scalp in areas stressed by combing, braiding, or sleeping."

The researchers suggest the following hair care tips and treatments:

- Use a well-trained professional for thermal and chemical procedures to help avoid damage.
- Limit hot comb treatments to once weekly, and make sure they are done on clean, dry hair.
- If hair is already damaged, it should be trimmed, and moisturizing shampoos and conditioners should be used.
- When undergoing chemical relaxation, the scalp should be protected through "scalp basing," a thick emollient used on the scalp to prevent skin irritation.
- Trim hair on a regular basis, and have chemical relaxation done no more than every six to eight weeks.
- Use of hair gels, sprays, and spritzes for hair sculpting can also lead to the condition. Less-damaging natural hairstyles, wigs, and moisturizing hair products should be considered.

Central centrifugal cicatricial alopecia in African American women is not clearly associated with hair care products. Black women with the condition should consider many of the same recommendations as above when undergoing chemical relaxation. A "relaxer holiday," as well as a natural, chemical-free hairstyle, might be considered.

Traction alopecia is particularly common among African American women, and treatment involves changing the hairstyle that is causing the trauma. If folliculitis is present, oral or topical antibiotics may be prescribed. If there is inflammation, treatment may be similar to that for alopecia areata, with use of either topical or intralesional (injected into the bald areas) corticosteroids. "In the present authors' practice, topical minoxidil as a treatment for traction alopecia has been found to be a successful option for some patients," Callender writes.

Seborrheic dermatitis may be a problem for African American women, again sometimes resulting from hair care techniques and products.

Some recommendations for this condition are:

- Therapeutic shampoos containing ciclopirox and zinc pyrithione are especially good for women who chemically straighten their hair.
- Other over-the-counter antidandruff shampoos may be used in selected patients, but they should not be used daily, as the labels suggest they can cause excessive dryness or breakage.
- Read labels. Therapeutic shampoos containing tar, selenium sulfide, and salicylic acid may be harsh on chemically treated hair.

While there is no difference in the manifestation of female pattern hair loss in black women, it should be noted that the use of topical minoxidil can result in undoing the effect of chemical straightening, rendering the hair back to its naturally curly state. "While not commonly found, compounding pharmacies can provide the patients with minoxidil in an ointment base as an alternative vehicle that is more compatible with their hairstyle," Callender writes.

8

Ironing out Ferritin

One topic that often comes up on many Internet hair loss help forums, and in many articles on the subject, is the possible association between iron levels and loss of hair. The fact that nearly every woman who wrote to me was either taking or considering taking iron supplementation prompted me to devote an entire chapter to this issue. I was curious to find out if there was a clear link or just a presumptive association between low iron levels and hair loss.

"It's interesting—most women, by the time they reach menopause, have some degree of iron deficiency, and it may be a contributing factor to hair loss, but it's not the whole story," Wendel says. "And that's what I usually tell my patients. Yes, we need to make sure that your iron levels are good, because [iron deficiency] could make your hair loss happen faster, and I've seen that in a variety of patients, but the reality is that they need to have a complete medical evaluation, and part of that evaluation is to check the iron levels."

According to medical experts, women who are most at risk for low iron levels include premenopausal women (especially those with heavy or frequent periods), vegetarians, women who crash diet, women who suffer from anorexia or bulimia, and those who exercise heavily (to the point of the cessation of menstruation).

Ferritin Levels

When looking at iron deficiency, doctors are often looking at your ferritin levels. This is not the amount of circulating iron but the amount of iron your body has stored for future use.

Haber told me that iron deficiency is "the number one thing that I discover in all the labs that I do—some kind of abnormality, either in women's iron stores, ferritin levels, or true anemia, and I correct that." He says after the iron levels are corrected, some women have a slowdown in their hair loss, but correcting iron levels is not solving everyone's problem.

"If you looked at one hundred women with hair loss and checked for anemia and checked one hundred women without hair loss, you're probably going to find a subtle anemia in both groups. No one has done that study, but I suspect that they might both be the same."

Jeffrey Miller, M.D., a board-certified dermatologist with Penn State College of Medicine in Hershey, Pennsylvania, said the issue with iron levels is very confusing and noted the lack of well-controlled studies showing that replacing iron improves hair loss.

In the studies that have been done, as well as in the wealth of anecdotal evidence both pro and con for iron replacement and hair loss, there does not appear to be any clear consensus on the issue.

Clinical Studies on Hair Loss and Ferritin

One study conducted by Janet L. Roberts, M.D., of Oregon Health Sciences University in Portland, Oregon, looked at 153 women who had been diagnosed with TE and were either premenopausal or postmenopausal. After ruling out women who had FPHL or other factors as the cause, she concluded that 72 percent of the premenopausal women had iron deficiency as the cause of their TE. However, she also discovered that 49 percent of the postmenopausal women suffered from drug-induced TE. Nonetheless, Roberts concluded that while "medications are the most common cause of telogen effluvium in postmenopausal women, iron deficiency should not be ruled out."

Moreover, there appears to be a wide "normal" range for ferritin levels (12 to 150 ng/ml [nanograms per millileter]), according to MedlinePlus from the National Institutes of Health's National Library of Medicine. The United Kingdom's National Health Services uses 20 to 200 ng/ml as normal. Iron deficiency may be present, the NIH and NHS say, at the lower end of the range. An article in *Environmental Nutrition* in 2004 noted that in women, ferritin levels lower than 40 ng/ml may be associated with hair loss; however, some women continue to experience TE with ferritin levels at 70 or greater.

I found it difficult to find a clear cause-and-effect relationship between ferritin levels and hair loss, or even specifically between ferritin levels and TE, in the medical literature. A lot of the study has been either observational (Roberts's study was a chart review) or anecdotal, containing various reports of patients who were found to be anemic and had hair loss.

A small study from the University of Pennsylvania School of Medicine, which compared women with various types of hair loss to a similar group of women without hair loss (dubbed "normals"), found that mean ferritin levels in women with TE and alopecia totalis were not significantly lower than the levels in the women without hair loss, but those with FPHL and alopecia areata had lower ferritin levels that were statistically significant. The researchers concluded: "Our findings have implications regarding therapeutics, clinical trial design, and understanding the triggers for alopecia." This means ferritin levels might indeed play a role in FPHL. But again, this is a small study with only 117 participants and in no way rules out entirely ferritin's role in TE. It just means that ferritin levels need to be taken into account as part of the entire differential diagnosis in determining why your hair is falling out.

But wait, there's more.

An Australian study decided to take a crack at this ferritin-hair loss relationship as well. The study included 194 women who, between 1997 and 1999, visited a specialist hair clinic with diffuse TE of six months' or greater duration. They were screened and tested to determine if they had TE or FPH. The laboratory the researchers used for the study designated 20 as the low limit of normal for ferritin levels, and that cutoff point was used for the study.

Androgenetic alopecia was found in 117 (60 percent) of the participants. Minoxidil was not used in any of the patients in the study, but those who were diagnosed as having androgenetic alopecia were given either 200 milligrams of spironolactone daily or 100 milligrams of cyproterone acetate daily for ten days each month.

Only twelve of the patients had a serum ferritin of 20 or less, and seven of them were diagnosed on biopsy as having FPHL, with the remainder having a differential diagnosis of primary chronic telogen effluvium and chronic telogen hair loss, secondary to iron deficiency. These twelve patients were given oral iron supplements for a minimum of three months.

Those patients who were found to still have a serum ferritin lower than 20 were kept on iron supplementation for another three months. Four patients fell in this category. After six months, all the patients had serum ferritin levels above 20.

Seven of the patients who were given iron supplementation were also given spironolactone. Of these, four experienced a reduction of hair shedding and an increase in hair volume over a six-month period, while there was no change in hair density, a result similar to that in the other 108 patients who received the oral anti-androgen therapy (spironolactone) for androgenetic alopecia. So the study is actually inconclusive as to ferritin's role alone.

Taking Iron Supplementation for Hair Loss

Nonetheless, it does seem that having optimal iron stores is important and may indeed play a part in keeping your hair healthy. Does that mean you should take iron supplementation? Possibly. Ask your doctor to test for it, especially if you suffer with heavy menstrual periods or have had a recent blood loss or an operation.

However, make sure you know your complete iron profile before simply taking megadoses of iron, as too much iron can have profound consequences.

At the very least, iron supplementation can cause constipation, which is a common side effect, but if you overdo it, you could be prone to iron overload, which will damage your liver. You'd have to take a lot of iron to do this, but as with anything, if you think you need megadoses of iron or any other vitamin, mineral, or herb, it's best to discuss this with a nutritionist, doctor, or medical specialist well-versed in supplementation. Some alternative-medicine practitioners—such as holistic practitioners, chiropractors, and naturopaths—have expertise in this area as well.

According to the Institute of Medicine's Food Nutrition Board, a female from age fourteen to eighteen needs a

Assessing Study Claims

When looking at scientific studies, pay attention to their design. Stronger studies look at women with hair loss and a control group of women without hair loss culled from similar demographics. Other strong hair studies, particularly those assessing efficacy of topical treatments, are "half-head" studies in which, just as it sounds, the product is only applied to one half of the head and the two sections are compared over a certain time. If a systemic treatment, such as a pill, is being tried, look for a blinded, placebo-controlled study. This means that one part of the group is being given a dummy pill without their knowledge, making the assessment of the trial's results fairly objective.

Epidemiological studies, or those that look at populations, may offer some good information, especially if conducted in a large population and/or over a long period of time.

Be wary, however, of studies that have only a small number of participants, are conducted without a control group, or are funded by a drug, device, or supplement company. Company funding may not necessarily lead to a bad study design, but you should be able to find other studies without company ties that corroborate the findings.

daily intake of 15 milligrams of iron; from age nineteen to fifty, 18 milligrams; and after age fifty, 8 milligrams.

"Generally, I tell my patients to take a good multivitamin with just a little bit of iron in it," Wendel told me. She notes that vitamins labeled for women over fifty do not contain iron "because they assume that once you stop getting your period, you don't need it anymore, so be careful to get a little iron supplement as well."

9

Hair Nutrients

Lots of people talk about the possibility of certain vitamin deficiencies causing hair loss. If eating right were the crux of the problem many of us suffering from hair loss would be cured and most fast-food junkies would be bald. Alas, this is another idea that doesn't hold water across the board, but that doesn't mean taking supplements and eating well aren't important, it's just not the be-all and end-all of hair loss.

Still, if your diet isn't optimal, your hair could suffer, so a discussion of vitamin, mineral, nutrient, and herbal supplementation is certainly in order with the following caveat: Unlike pharmaceutical products, supplements often don't undergo rigorous clinical testing. This is slowly changing as the popularity of alternative medicines is driving the industry to uniformity (see Appendix B), but you need to use a certain amount of caution when taking any supplement for your hair, whether or not it is deemed "natural."

Biotin and Folic Acid: The Dynamic Duo for Hair Health

Biotin and folic acid (vitamin B9, folate) are considered the two essential vitamins for hair health. But rarely is anyone deficient in them, as they are readily obtained through a well-balanced diet.

The recommended daily allowance (RDA) for folic acid for women is 400 mcg (micrograms); for women who are pregnant or lactating, the RDA is 600 mcg.

Possible side effects: If folic acid supplementation exceeds 1,000 mcg per day, it can trigger the symptoms of vitamin B12 deficiency. Untreated B12 deficiency can, even if corrected, result in permanent nerve damage, according to the U.S. Office of Dietary Supplements.

Nutritional sources of folic acid include orange juice, spinach, fortified breakfast cereals, tomato juice, whole grains, bananas, and cantaloupe.

The usual suggested amount of daily biotin is 300 mcg, although there is no actual established RDA for the vitamin. Biotin deficiency has been shown in people who consume large amounts of raw egg whites and people who have malabsorption syndromes who are undergoing parenteral nutrition (tube feeding) without biotin supplementation.

My research found this contradiction with biotin use: One source noted that there have been no documented cases of biotin overdose, while another notes that too much biotin can cause hair loss! Stay within the recommended daily doses.

Possible side effects: Other than the above, I did not find any.

Food sources of biotin include liver, egg yolks, soybeans, clams, mushrooms, and bananas.

Zinc

Here's another contradiction I've found in the medical literature: Hair loss is a sign of zinc deficiency, but hair loss is also a sign of zinc overdose! Doesn't make you want to fool with it, does it?

The RDA for zinc for women over age nineteen is 8 mg (milligrams). If you are pregnant or lactating, the RDA is 11 mg and 12 mg, respectively.

Possible side effects: Taking 150 to 450 mg of zinc may result in a depressed immune system, poor wound healing, hair loss, and the inability to taste or smell. It can also block iron absorption, which has been established as being important for preventing hair loss for some. Food sources of zinc include oysters, red meat and poultry, nuts, certain seafood, whole grains, fortified breakfast cereals, and dairy products.

Vitamin A

Vitamin A (sometimes listed as beta carotene or vitamin A acetate) is, along with vitamins D, E, and K, a fat-soluble vitamin, meaning it is stored in the body for a long time, and therefore a cumulative buildup of toxic levels is possible. The RDA for vitamin A is listed as 700 mcg or 2,300 IU (International Units).

While vitamin A is important for your hair and skin, it is likely that you get plenty in your daily diet from foods such as liver, eggs, milk and cheese, carrots, cantaloupe, and spinach, as well as in most fortified cereals and in daily multivitamin supplements.

Possible side effects: Excess doses of vitamin A may cause birth defects, compromise bone health and the ability for blood to clot, and overstimulate the immune system.

Vitamins and Minerals Formulated for Hair

I wish I could point to a hair supplement and say, "Eureka! This will cure your woes!" But I cannot. Go into any health food store or online, and you will find plenty of vitamin and mineral supplements claiming to specifically target your hair's nutritional needs. Read the labels on these carefully, and compare them to regular multivitamins.

The table on the opposite page compares active ingredients in three sample hair vitamins and a popular multivitamin. As you will see, the formulations of the hair vitamins are fairly similar to that of the multivitamin, which also contains some key nutrients, such as calcium, that the hair vitamins do not.

I'm not saying that the hair vitamins are useless or harmful, but before you spend money on them, consider supplementing your regular multivitamin with some of the nutrients it lacks, since the "hair supplements" do not seem to include all the ingredients that a normal multivitamin contains, such as lutein, lycopene, calcium, magnesium, vitamins C and D, and some others.

Adding biotin and folic acid supplementation to your daily regimen might be the best path to take. Many women tell me that even though taking these two vitamins did not seem to regrow their hair, their hair and nails did seem to grow faster and stronger. Haber seems to concur. "I've used biotin and folic acid in an untold number of women, but no one has come back with a thick, full head of hair. But again, maybe it's just a tiny thing helping to hold onto a couple thousand hairs, but maybe it's worth it, maybe it's just slowing down the loss," he says. "Won't be able to prove that, but it's certainly worth it."

And, do consider this: If you are taking a hair vitamin formulation in addition to a daily multivitamin,

Table: Comparison of Hair Vitamins to Popular Multivitamin

(More than one number for some ingredients indicates a range among the three sample hair vitamins.)

Active Ingredients	Amount in Hair Vitamins	Amount in Multivitamin
folic acid	200–400 mcg	400 mcg
biotin	300–5,000 mcg	30 mcg
zinc	3–15 mg	15 mg
vitamin A	4,000–5,000 IU	3,500 IU
vitamin B5	50–100 mg	10 mg
iodine	150 mcg	150 mcg
vitamin B12	6–35 mcg	6 mcg
vitamin B2	2 mg	1.7 mg
thiamine	2 mg	1.5 mg
vitamin B6	2 mg	2 mg
selenium	50 mcg	20 mcg
choline	250 mg	None
bitartrate	None	None
inositol	125 mg	None
PABA	35 mg	None
copper	1 mg*	2 mg
iron	None	18 mg
other	borage (710 mg) millet and L-methionine (300 mg); herbs: green tea, grape seed extract, and ginkgo biloba (270 mg)*	several not found in hair vitamins: vitamin C, calcium, magnesium, lycopene, lutein, etc.

*Amounts found in one (not all) hair vitamins.

and eating a lot of fortified foods as well, you may be overdosing on some essential nutrients and even causing your hair loss.

Prenatal Vitamins

A lot of the women who wrote to me, and those who post on hair loss Web sites, tout the use of prenatal vitamins. In my research, however, I did not uncover anything to suggest prenatal vitamins are somehow recommended for hair loss, other than anecdotally. I suspect the reason for their popularity is due to the added folic acid (which is important in preventing birth defects such as spina bifida) and to the fact that our hair is often so much healthier during pregnancy.

But is our hair healthier because of the vitamins or the pregnancy?

Remember, our hair's anagen phase is prolonged during pregnancy, so there is a cessation of hair shedding, and our hair appears (and indeed is, for that time) thicker than usual. However, once we give birth, our hair cycle

Count 'Em Up!

Read the labels on bottles of vitamins and minerals, and do the math! Remember, some vitamins in excess can be toxic, and some may even cause hair loss. Go to the Office of Dietary Supplement's Web site (http://ods.od.nih.gov), and look for fact sheets on particular supplements. Further resources are included in the appendices of this book.

returns to normal with its normal shedding cycle. It's not the folic acid per se that kept our hair from shedding as much during pregnancy, but the hormonal response and the interruption of our hair cycle.

I doubt there is anything wrong with taking prenatal vitamins when not pregnant, but talk with your physician about their potential to help with hair loss. Again, be sure to monitor your overall intake of vitamins and minerals to ensure you stay within the RDAs, which should be listed on the labels. Also check out this book's appendix for helpful information on dietary and other supplements.

Other Nutrients That May Help Your Hair

In addition to the supplements listed above, www. holisticonline.com, a good source for information on natural medicines, lists B6, inositol, pantothenic acid (B5), and niacin (B3), as well as the minerals magnesium and sulfur, as being important for hair health. The Web site also emphasizes the importance of essential fatty acids (such as flaxseed oil), evening primrose oil, salmon oil, vitamin E, and vitamin C; it even suggests the addition of raw thymus gland. I would not recommend using the latter unless you are under a physician's or naturopath's care (and, ideally, seeing both, who are talking with each other).

The supplements the Web site recommends can mostly be obtained through your diet, but if you choose to supplement, be mindful of the recommended RDAs, and do not exceed the maximum recommended dosage unless directed by a physician to do so.

Use Supplements with Caution

You'll see a lot of nutrients touted for hair loss, from the benign suggestion to drink green tea to taking a gammolinolenic acid such as evening primrose oil. Some of these ingredients are included in the hair formulations listed above. HerAlopecia.com and HairLossTalk.com offer a list of diet and dietary supplements, and both Web sites are probably a good place to start to determine if you want to try them. Both offer this advice: Consider supplements as complementary treatments helping to give you optimal health. HerAlopecia.com also says that you need to allow four to eight weeks to see results from a nutritional change, so be patient.

But remember: The word "natural" doesn't automatically mean "safe." If you take any supplements, you should do so with the same amount of care you would take when using over-the-counter or prescription medicines.

These things can be powerful stuff.

For instance, evening primrose oil is suggested as a remedy for a number of ailments—psoriasis, rheumatoid arthritis, breast pain and breast cysts, and the symptoms of menopause, as well as hair loss. There is not a large body of scientific evidence for these and other claims, even though there is a wealth of anecdotal and historic evidence. Nonetheless, according to the Aetna Intelihealth Web site, people with seizures or who are allergic to plants in the Onagraceae family should avoid taking it. Other side effects may include headache, stomach pain, nausea, and loose stools. Seizures might also occur if taken with phenothiazine drugs such as Thorazine.

My purpose here is not to say such treatments do not work or to dissuade you from taking them, but to get you to think before you ingest. My experience and research has led me to one very large worry—that women, myself included, will try just about anything to stop their hair loss.

A Hair Loss Diet?

A lot of books on the subject of hair loss also include a chapter on nutrition. The main thing about eating well and hair loss is that you don't want to be yo-yo dieting, having your weight go up and down—no rapid weight loss, in other words. Many of the women who wrote to me have suffered from bulimia or anorexia, as is common in our thinness-obsessed society. These extreme eating disorders can have an adverse effect on your hair, as they can deplete your body of many of the important nutrients listed above.

Wendel advises a commonsense diet with complex carbohydrates to keep your metabolism on a steady level, while avoiding high-sugar snacks. I questioned her about sugar intake: "I don't think there's a direct correlation between high sugar [intake] and hair loss; a good diet is really an effort to get women to think more carefully about their diet and to eat a well-balanced diet," she told me.

So, really, there is no "hair loss diet," per se. Know your body, talk to your doctor if you are overweight, and ask to have a dietitian help work out a healthful, well-balanced weight-loss plan—one with your hair in mind!

Remember: plenty of anorexic and bulimic women do not lose their hair. Lots of people eat all the wrong things and yet have a wonderful head of hair and somehow also remain disease-free.

My theory is that those of us who are prone to hair loss must make every effort to be as optimally healthy as possible. It is my opinion that for us, our hair is our Achilles heel and the barometer for our overall health. So eat well, and exercise regularly. Being healthy is important for more than just our hair, and while it may not help grow more hair, it probably will help us better maintain what we have.

10

Lasers, Volumizers, Cover–Ups, and Wigs

The Laser Comb: Help or Hype?

There's a lot of buzz about the HairMax laser comb, manufactured by Lexington International of Boca Raton, Florida. David Michaels, one of the developers of the comb, which looks like a bionic hairbrush, told me the device is "a well-founded hope in the fight against hair loss."

I will admit my skepticism.

One small clinical study, conducted by John L. Satino and Michael Markou, D.O., of the Laser Hair and Scalp Clinic in Clearwater, Florida, tested the laser comb in thirty-five patients (twenty-eight men, seven women) with androgenetic alopecia for six months. They tested hair strength and did hair counts in the areas where the participants had the greatest amount of hair loss. Their results were quite impressive—hair counts increased on average by 93.5 percent, and hair strength showed a 78.9 percent increase in all patients.

But this is just one very small study.

The laser comb's developers point to the fact that low-level laser light therapy (LLLT), the mechanism the comb uses, has had a good track record since the 1960s as a treatment for wound healing. "LLLT is starting to become recognized in North America as an effective modality for alopecia and other dermatological medical conditions," said Martin Unger, M.D., a recognized authority on hair restoration and medical director of Lexington International.

In the United States, the HairMax laser comb is only approved for safety, meaning that it won't hurt you and is safe to use, but not that it will necessarily regrow hair. However, in Canada it is "certified as a class 2 medical device for claims and indications to strengthen hair, prevent hair loss and stimulate regrowth of scalp hair in men and women."

I truly expected most of the physicians I spoke with to debunk the laser comb, but I was surprised.

"I love the thought of it," Wendel told me when I asked her opinion of it. She pointed to the same study I relayed here and spoke of the incredible results. She says she tells patients that if money is not a factor, it's worth a try.

Jerry Cooley, M.D., a board-certified dermatologist in hair restoration with a private practice at the Carolina Dermatology Hair Center in Charlotte, North Carolina, says he tells his patients about the laser comb and has seen some of them benefit from it. "It makes more of what you have," he says. "The laser comb is one more complementary thing, but there is no one miracle product."

Some of the women who wrote to me have bought the comb, and others are saving their pennies to purchase it. No one has said it has regrown their hair, but they do report that their hair looks better—thicker and fuller.

Neil Saddick, M.D., FACP, a clinical professor and attending physician in the department of dermatology at New York Hospital, Cornell University, took a more moderate stance on the laser technology and told me, "It's too early to tell; needs further testing."

The laser comb is pricey; at the time this book was written, its cost was listed as $625 (see http://www.lasercomb.net/theStore.html). LLLT is also used in salons; six months of treatment can cost upward of $3,000.

The laser comb can be returned within twelve weeks if you are unsatisfied with the product for any reason, but I asked Michaels if this was really fair, considering it can take four to six months to see true hair regrowth. "We're not saying you will see dramatic benefits within twelve weeks," he said. "But certainly within twelve weeks you will see that hair is responding favorably to the laser energy. It's growing a little faster, less hair is falling out, and it's more manageable."

I also asked him, if the HairMax laser comb works so well, why isn't everyone using it? He replied, "We're staying pretty much low-key right now until we get FDA clearance. The medical community has not embraced us yet."

In my opinion, if you have the money to spend, go for it, but realize that so far, no one is reporting stellar hair regrowth using this product. However, it can be seen as another therapy in the armamentarium of products to use to make the most of what you have.

Volumizers and Cover-ups

The grocery and pharmacy aisles are bulging with hair care products. If you're like me, you've probably tried all of the products with the words "adds volume," "for fine or thinning hair," "improves the appearance of fine and thinning hair," or other such verbiage on the labels. This billion-dollar world of volumizing shampoos, conditioners, gels, mousses, and sprays are appealing to a large population, and if there weren't so many of us, men and

Hair Loss Myth #6

Shampooing causes hair loss.

Not true. Those who are losing their hair often wrongly believe that shampooing too often causes more hair to fall out. This may be because shedding is easier to notice when it collects in the drain, or because hair that is prone to shedding easily can come out with even a little extra traction. But the total amount of hair lost does not increase with normal shampooing. Hair that is dirty will often look duller and thinner, so it is best to follow the same routine as before hair loss began. Just use a mild shampoo and be easy on your scalp.

—*Anita Bhorjee*

women alike, seeking to have at least the appearance of thicker, fuller hair, you can bet they wouldn't exist. In the face of the incredible lack of truly viable treatments for hair loss, we dip into our pocketbooks on a regular basis and buy hope in a bottle.

There are so many products that to try to list them all and give an assessment or overview would be impossible. You'll find your hair really responds to some products, but not to others. None of them, however, will grow hair, with the possible exception of Nizoral shampoo, which, as stated before contains, ketoconazole.

Camouflage Products

Some products get right to the chase and claim only to help you cover up your hair loss. They are, in my mind, at least honest about it. Camouflage products give the appearance of more hair either by coloring the scalp to match your hair color or by using sprayed-on fibers to give the illusion of more hair.

Since there are always new products in this realm coming on the market, I suggest you check them out on a credible hair loss Web site such as HairLossTalk.com, HerAlopecia.com, or one of the other Web sites I list in Appendix A.

Two camouflage products that seem to have the best track records are Toppik and Couvré. Toppik uses microfibers that bind onto your hair and, according to HairLossTalk.com, stay in place for twenty-four hours and are not affected by wind or rain. The product is removed upon shampooing, however.

Couvré does not contain any fibers; it's a lotion that is applied to the scalp to help with "see-through" hair. According to HairLossTalk.com, the product has been recommended for use by dermatologists and is safe. Couvré and Toppik used together provide greater camouflage and work nicely for some people.

Wearing Hair: The Treatment of Last Resort

Wearing additional hair, like using camouflage products, is the bend in the road none of us wants to come to when discussing hair loss solutions—they are treatments of last resort. But you may find that wearing hair, at least on occasion, can help with those social situations you might otherwise avoid, or can help bolster your self-esteem as you are trying various medical treatments or undergoing a transplant.

The American Hair Loss Council (www.ahlc.org) is a good place to start for information on hair additions, wigs, hair weaves, etc. While the organization does not endorse a particular salon or individual who works in this area, its members do agree to honor the organization's code of ethics, and the Web site has a listing of its specialists by geographic location.

Hair additions, the AHLC says, are the safest way to gain hair. There are only two procedures the council does not recommend—sutures and tunnel grafts. These procedures are invasive surgical procedures and can cause infection and other complications.

In general, hair additions are attached either to existing hair or to the skin. Those procedures using existing hair are often called weaves, cabling, fusion, microlinks, bonding, and beading. Through various procedures, hair additions are attached to existing hair and must be reapplied or tightened as the existing hair grows.

Added hair may also be attached to the skin through the use of adhesives, either two-sided tape or a special glue-like liquid. Suction through the use of form-fitting caps can also be used.

There are some caveats—which the AHLC outlines—to using these forms of hair enhancements:

- Although most adhesives are safe, it is best to have a patch test done by a dermatologist if you have a history of allergies. Even if you do not, it's always best to have a patch test done in advance.
- Hair weaving and other types of attachments that involve prolonged tension can cause permanent hair loss at the anchor site on fine, thin hair. (Even temporary clips attached too tightly can cause permanent hair loss.) When performed properly on the qualified client, hair weaving does not cause hair loss.
- Proper hygiene must be maintained when wearing a hair addition for extended periods of time. It is essential that one must clean the scalp and hair on a regular basis.

Hair additions don't come cheaply. The AHLC says they can range in price from $750 to $2,500. They can consist of either synthetic or human hair.

Check out the qualifications of the salon you are visiting for any type of hair attachment, and be sure to talk with your physician to see if this is an option for your type of hair loss or if it has the potential to cause more damage.

Wigs

Those of us experiencing hair loss are asked, if all other options fail, to pick out a selection of pretty hats and scarves or a nice wig. Even many of the doctors I spoke with, after detailing the various causes and possible treatments for hair loss, gave the option of a wig with little hesitation, as if it's not a big deal.

Telling a woman who is just coming to grips with the fact that she is losing her hair about the nice wigs available nowadays is nearly as insensitive as telling an infertile couple, "Well, you can always adopt." This is not a decision to come to easily, and it is the treatment or nontreatment of last resort. A woman coming to terms with her hair loss has a completely different mindset from a woman with hair who decides to try on wigs as a fun hair option.

Experts say that when you do find the wig you like, you should take it to your hairdresser to have it customized for you. Wigs right off the rack often have enough hair for three people. Get it thinned, cut, and styled for your face; otherwise it will look fake.

Spend time, not money, finding a hair system or wig.

Hair Extensions and Additions

Where wigs are fairly benign and cannot hurt the hair you have, hair additions and extensions have the potential to cause problems and could end up damaging the hair you have left.

Hair Loss Myth #7

Chemical hair products cause hair loss.

Not true—if they are used with care. In 1994, the FDA warned patients to stop using hair relaxer products made by the company World Rio Corporation after it received over 3,000 complaints of negative results including hair loss and scalp irritation. In general, however, relaxers, permanents, and hair dyes are generally safe for the scalp and hair with some caveats: Stick with well-known brands, do not exceed time limits given in the directions (longer application does not lead to better results), do a patch test if recommended to guard against allergic reaction, and do not apply two types of treatments, such as color and wave, in the same week. Chemicals are never easy on your hair, but used with a little caution, they allow you to play magician with the hair nature gave you.

—*Anita Bhorjee*

Use caution if you are considering extensions. Ask your salon if their hairdressers are experienced in working with people who are losing their hair (as opposed to those who simply want to enhance the normal amount of hair they already have) and whether you can speak with their other clients with hair similar to yours. Again, go to the AHLC Web site to find a specialist who has agreed to that group's code of ethics for working with hair additions and systems.

11

Tracking the Hair Loss Holy Grail

While I wish I could point to one treatment and say, "This is the Holy Grail for hair loss," I cannot. No one can.

But, like you, I keep searching. I am ashamed to admit that even with my knowledge culled from years of being a medical journalist, I am easily susceptible to the promise of a cure.

One night I couldn't sleep, and even with more than one hundred channels to choose from on my satellite television service, all I could find to watch were infomercials. One caught my attention—an inversion table. At first, because I suffer with arthritis in my neck resulting from a fall from a horse as a child, I wondered if it might help my chronic neck pain.

But here's what really made me sit up and take notice—a viewer phoned in and endorsed the product by saying, "It is even helping me regrow my hair!"

I was fully awake at that point.

A Fool and Hair Money Are Soon Parted

The moderators, of course, quickly said they couldn't make such claims. But it was a done deal—I was pulling my credit card out of my wallet, and within a few weeks the inversion table arrived at my home. Some odd, convoluted logic, probably coupled with sleep deprivation, said this might just be the answer to my prayers.

No, of course it has not helped my hair.

However, it has helped my neck. Nonetheless, it's a monster sitting in my bedroom attesting to my gullibility, my desire for even a modest glimmer of hope that something could be a little-known miracle cure for my hair loss. And I write about medical issues for a living!

Many of the women who wrote to me admitted to trying nearly anything to grow their hair, some based on folk remedies, some simply born of desperation. These include: a paste made from cayenne pepper and water; doing headstands to improve blood flow (cheaper than the inversion table, at least); birth-control pills crushed into a powder added to shampoo (expensive shampoo!); zinc and vitamin B6 dissolved in water with lemon juice; egg; Indian herbs; a mixture of watercress, aloe gel, rosemary, and flax seed . . . and the list goes on. One woman said that at one point she was taking more than ten different nutrients!

Self-diagnosing and self-medicating can be costly and possibly dangerous, even if the medication is a vitamin or an herb, or a handful of vitamins and herbs. But I think we all do this because there seems to be a lack of support, both medically and emotionally, for our plight in dealing with hair loss. And despite the list of possible treatments I just outlined for the condition, none seems to work very well or for very long.

Treatment Talk

That said, let's talk a bit about the real-world use of some of these treatments.

Like it or not (and many of the women who wrote to me hate it), topical minoxidil (Rogaine) is the standard treatment for hair loss.

"It is really the best thing out there for women. It works by mechanisms we don't quite understand, treating a disease we don't understand, with a drug we don't understand, which is perhaps odd, but we know it works, it's fairly benign, and we don't have anything better or safer," Haber told me. He says that no matter the type of hair loss, he prescribes the treatment for every woman he sees in his practice, "because it can slow the process, no matter what's happening."

Wendel says that probably fewer than 20 percent of the patients in her practice see hair regrowth with topical minoxidil. "But most get a longer growth phase, they shed less, and they will hold onto their hair longer. I'm not suggesting it's going to stop the progress completely, but anything that can slow down the process is definitely worth doing," she told me.

And this alone may be a decent enough reason to stick with a daily minoxidil regimen.

Beware of the Knee-Jerk Rogaine Response

But beware if Rogaine is the first and only option presented to you when you bring up your hair loss with your physician. For many doctors, the automatic response to hair loss is all Rogaine, all the time. It's kind of the physician's Stepford-wife-like response: Hair loss? Rogaine. Yes, but . . . perhaps there's another cause/treatment . . . . Hair loss? Rogaine.

This is the attitude that Lori, thirty-five, encountered. She was told to reduce her stress and use Rogaine, with little other tests or a clear diagnosis. She says she's been using Rogaine for several months and has not seen any change so far.

Topical minoxidil should be the treatment option you're left with after you've had a thorough evaluation of your particular hair loss situation.

Sure, it's the mainstay of treatment, but given that, for most of us, at best it will allow us to keep what little we have, it certainly shouldn't be handed out as if it's some magical elixir.

"I've used Rogaine for almost a year, and I haven't noticed any worsening," Shelly, twenty-five, wrote to me. "I have noticed some fine, thin hairs, but I don't think these hairs improve my hair cosmetically."

Kris, thirty-eight, gives this advice about Rogaine: "The main thing is patience. It took a year or more to see real results. So you cannot expect a miracle in a week or month."

Others tried it and couldn't cope with the greasiness or messiness of it, and some gave up after not seeing any results. Melinda says she has been using Rogaine for three years and saw a lot of improvement in the first year, but after two years it seemed to stop working, and "now my hair is atrophying again."

And then there is the problem of having to use topical minoxidil on a twice-daily basis. The routine gets a bit tiresome and expensive.

"I'm not comfortable making a lifetime commitment to Rogaine. I'm in my twenties and didn't want to pour a drug on my head for the rest of my life," Mary, twenty-seven, says. She echoes the opinion of many other women who wrote to me. Minoxidil is not easy, and it is a lifetime commitment—at least until something better comes along. This is difficult for young women. I didn't begin using it until I entered menopause at age fifty-three, and already I'm getting bored with it.

Tip: Take Pictures of Your Hair

It's difficult to see subtle improvements in hair growth. Remember, it takes three to six months to see new hair growth. So take some pictures of your scalp before you begin your treatment regimen, and then more photos at intervals of three months, six months, and a year. Often dermatologists will do this as well. This way, you have an objective tool for gauging whether you're gaining any benefit from a treatment. Yes, improvement can be that subtle.

But if it seems, at the very least, to be helping you hold on to what you have, especially if you're also using other therapies, it may be worth sticking with. I think of it the way I'd think about taking medication for high blood pressure or insulin for diabetes—it's all I have while waiting for a better treatment or a cure.

Using Other Hair Loss Treatments

But while so many of the women who wrote to me were skeptical of using something relatively safe like Rogaine, there seemed to be few expressed safety concerns about other medications, such as spironolactone or even Propecia, other than concerns about pregnancy.

Melissa, forty, says she found Rogaine too messy to use and is now taking Tagamet and 25 milligrams of spironolactone for her hair loss, but she is not seeing any results. She questions whether the 25-milligram dose of spironolactone is too low. It's likely, as stated before, that 200 milligrams per day is needed to see results, but, of course, that comes with more adverse side effects. I question the use of a systemic drug if there are no visible results. But even so-called natural treatments can have bad side effects.

Rhani had been using topical minoxidil for eight years. It seemed to be helping, even though it did not stop the incessant shedding associated with her chronic telogen effluvium. Nonetheless, she decided to take a break from the treatment and try saw palmetto. She says the herb "seemed like the answer to my prayers. The shedding calmed way down, but after about six months I began having an awful side effect. My periods got painful for the first time in my life, and my endometrium did not shed properly during my periods." Rhani ended up having a D & C (dilatation and curettage) to remove the excess tissue from her uterus. "When I stopped the saw palmetto, everything returned to normal."

After doing her own research, Rhani decided that spironolactone might work for her. Her condition is also marked by a lot of acne. She got an appointment with an endocrinologist, who agreed to prescribe the medication for her. She has noticed some new hair growth, and her acne has cleared, but the shedding still persists.

Sandra, fifty-six, is a breast cancer survivor. She is taking the aromatase inhibitor Arimidex to prevent her cancer from returning and is having problems with hair thinning. She wonders if other women taking this drug are having the same problems. I looked up information on the drug, and hair loss is listed as a possible side effect, and since aromatase keeps DHT at bay, hair loss from using an aromatase inhibitor makes sense. However, if you are taking this drug, do not stop taking it, as it's very important for preventing the return of the cancer. However, do speak with your oncologist and dermatologist or endocrinologist about your concerns about hair loss for advice on possibly thwarting this particular side effect. "If it's cancer or thin hair," Sandra says, "I will take thin hair. I am not happy about my hair, but I am alive and well. I hope my body will adjust and my hair will return."

I am concerned, however, that not everyone has Sandra's calm attitude toward hair loss and treatments and side effects. In reading hair loss Web sites, I have become increasingly worried about the quest for drugs to help control hair loss, and it appears some people are ordering treatments such as spironolactone, possibly without bona fide physicians' prescriptions or supervision, from Internet pharmacies. If you are doing this or considering doing this, please reconsider. Systemic treatments do not just go to your hair but can bring with them serious side effects.

Talk with your physician. If you wish to try a treatment and he or she doesn't think it's viable for your situation, but your research has you convinced you want to try it, at least elicit your doctor's help and guidance, as Rhani did, to try it for a certain period of time. This may not be easy, but it is better to seek out another doctor to oversee the treatments you want to try than to self-medicate and then need treatment for adverse side effects.

Wigged Out

Some of the women who wrote have chosen to wear hair rather than deal with the cost and side effects of topical or systemic treatments. They shared their frustrations and tips for choosing wigs and extensions with me.

Barbara purchased a $1,600 hairpiece that attached with clips when her hair loss first began. She feels it was "a complete rip-off and a scam. I wore it maybe five times. I then purchased some synthetic wigs. I have thrown out three of them and kept one. My next purchases were human-hair custom wigs." She suggests starting with synthetic wigs "to get used to wearing them, as they are less expensive." She notes they will fit differently depending on how much of your own hair you have. "I would suggest finding the lightest weight with a breathable cap. Wigs can get very uncomfortable in hot weather."

She says she hasn't worn them in windy weather and no longer wears them all the time. "I now personally choose not to wear them unless I am going someplace that I just feel too uncomfortable without a cover." A lot of women said they feel this way.

Melinda, thirty, wrote to me very upset about hair additions she had put in. She says she went with a very popular brand that was touted as being safe for women with fine, thinning hair. "It's supposed to be our 'answer,' and it's true it gives you more body. I had it done two weeks ago, but boy, was I in for a huge surprise! It has pulled my hair out by the root everywhere I had them put in, probably from the traction." She is concerned that removing them will make her hair far worse than before she had the extensions put in.

Frankie had tried hair extensions when her hair first began thinning but did not have a good experience with them. "They added thickness to my hair and I was so very proud of them, but after a few attempts, I realized that they were only contributing to the problem and making my hair even thinner. At the time, this was a very depressing experience."

Fran, thirty-six, sums up the "to wear hair or not to wear hair" question this way: "I wish our society made it easier for women to just go bald when faced with hair loss rather than expend so much time, energy, and money on creating the illusion of hair. Most sources focus on where to buy a wig, or how to tie a scarf. This information should be available for those who want it, but sources often assume women will cover up their hair loss and inadvertently imply that they should."

What the Future May Hold

It breaks my heart that this is not the largest section of this book. There is research going on in hair and baldness, with the majority being undertaken by the National Alopecia Areata Foundation and Duvic and her colleagues at M. D. Anderson, but hair research is certainly not at or near the top of many research agendas.

Still, every so often discovery of certain hair genes makes headlines—the Sonic Hedgehog gene, the Frizzled 6 gene—but these early animal studies are far from ready for prime time. Nonetheless, it's good to know that researchers at Columbia University's Hair and Research Center, the University of Pennsylvania, Johns Hopkins School of Medicine, the Howard Hughes Medical Institute, and other centers are on the early frontier of trying to zero in on the cause of baldness and its eventual cure.

Stem Cell Research

Researchers in Lausanne, Switzerland, are looking at the long-term renewal of hair follicles from stem cells. Their research, still in early-stage animal study, could eventually yield important information for hair growth. It's a long way from a rat study to humans, so keep an eye on this research, but don't hold your breath, especially given that stem cell research is a political and moral hot button right now.

Send in the Clones

While there have been rumors floating around that hair cloning is being done in Europe and that there have even been "hair banks" set up, as of this writing, we're not there yet. Nonetheless, this is probably the one new remedy that is on the near horizon.

Some exciting progress is being made in what is called follicular cell implantation, which some people refer to as "hair follicle cloning," "follicular neogenesis," "follicular regeneration," and "hair multiplication."

Jerry Cooley, M.D., along with his private practice at the Carolina Dermatology Hair Center, is a consultant for Intercytex, a tissue engineering company that is developing a follicular cell implantation treatment. He explained that the process is based on the idea of taking one hair from a person's donor site and transforming, or growing, it into one hundred or one thousand hairs in a petri dish, then transplanting those into the recipient site. So rather than having a one-to-one hair transplant, you have a one-to-one-thousand.

"If we have a way of overcoming the lack of donor hair, we have found the Holy Grail to hair loss," Cooley says.

Follicular cell implantation is being explored at various research centers around the globe, including Intercytex and the Aderans Research Institute (ARI), which is associated with Bosley Medical Center. "We have a staff of scientists at ARI that are not working on anything else," Washenik told me. At ARI, the process goes by the name "follicle neogenesis."

"It's incredibly exciting," Washenik says. "With each passing year, instead of there being more and more snake oil treatments, there are more and more real options, which is what is driving people to look at what is available to them now." He says taking advantage of the best treatments for hair loss now sets the stage for being ready for the next best treatment on the horizon when it becomes available.

While not yet ready for prime time, follicular cell implantation certainly appears to have a good shot at being perfected in the not-too-distant future: Cooley figures about ten years, while Washenik is more optimistic, predicting about five years. Let's hope it's sooner than later. But note, just before this book went to press, in an article in the *New Yorker* magazine Washenik said that if hair neogenesis does become a reality, it will likely go through the same evolution as hair transplantation did—looking very odd in the beginning and taking some time, possibly decades, to achieve a natural look.

12

Silent No More

The most difficult aspect of living with hair loss is coming to the realization that there is nothing left to try. If you've built a good hair loss team and yet there is little or no improvement, you will have to make some decisions and not let hair loss rule your life.

While you may have to concede a temporary defeat, make it clear to your physician and those around you that you want to continue to periodically evaluate your situation, especially in light of the possibility of new treatments coming on the horizon.

In the meantime you're left with possibly hanging on to what little you have with a treatment or two that at least doesn't make it worse.

Wendel and the other hair loss experts I spoke with told me that while there is no "cure" for FPHL or other types of hair loss that elude treatment, the goal is to control what you can control. "Not so long ago we wouldn't even think about women in terms of hair loss," Wendel points out, meaning that there wasn't even topical minoxidil or hair transplantation for women. So we've made some, albeit hardly many, gains.

She makes the following recommendations for women dealing with hair loss or who fear a worsening of their condition:

1. Eat a well-balanced diet with a combination of complex carbohydrates, protein, and some fat. Avoid high-sugar snacks.
2. If you need to lose weight, avoid crash diets, which can often cause or exacerbate hair loss. Follow only a doctor-recommended diet with no stimulants.
3. Take a multivitamin with a small amount of iron, especially during the childbearing years.
4. Learn to deal with stress better through meditation, yoga, and exercise.
5. Treat the hair you have gently by avoiding hair care products and methods that are harsh and can damage hair and its roots.
6. If you must color your hair, have it done professionally using products that do not contain peroxide or ammonia.
7. If you are a young woman on an oral contraceptive, make sure it is the type that can help rather than contribute to hair loss. If your hair is naturally thin, have an open discussion with your doctor before starting hormones.
8. If you are experiencing hair loss and have a family history of the problem, seek the help of a hair loss specialist at your first symptoms.
9. Have your hair styled and treated by professional stylists—they may be the first to notice a worsening (or an improvement!) of your condition.
10. Last and most important, get a yearly physical and have your doctor check you periodically for iron deficiency, hormonal imbalances, diabetes, and nutritional deficiencies, to make sure that these problems won't worsen your condition.

Whatever treatment or treatments you choose to try for controlling or stopping your hair loss, keep these points in mind:

- Take the treatments with a huge dose of patience. Because of hair-growth cycles, realize it will take as long as six months to a year to see any change.
- Have realistic expectations. Do not expect any treatment to give you more hair than you ever had, or even restore the hair you once had. Look for small changes, or work on maintaining what you have, so that anything above that is the icing on the cake.
- Watch for adverse side effects. Don't trade good health for your hair.
- Mention your hair loss to all your doctors to keep it on their radar.
- Check out any new treatment that appears on the Internet or in books and newspapers through a viable source—either a medical professional or some of the Web sites listed in Appendix A.
- Don't throw good money after bad hair treatments.
- And most of all, don't keep silent about women's hair loss. It's time we live it shame free.

Hair Loss Is a Loss with a Capital L

Like any other loss in your life, losing your hair is losing a part of you. It is a Loss, capital L.

To come to terms with balding, there has to be a process of letting go, just as there would be with any other loss—such as the loss of our youth.

Sooner or later, no matter what cosmetic procedures we can afford, age will catch up with us. We will not be able to fend off the fact that our youth is gone. We either emerge on the other side of the transition with a new-found perspective on the world, or we cross over feeling ravaged and bitter—exemplifying the worst aspects of age, rather than the best: acceptance, renewal of where we are in life, and contentment.

But age happens to us all, even to the Botoxed, lifted, and siliconed. Hair loss does not, which makes letting go even more difficult.

The mourning process for the loss of our hair is the same for mourning any death or dealing with any illness or condition. Elisabeth Kübler-Ross, who wrote the ground-breaking book *On Death and Dying*, lists five stages of grief. I found these on a cancer survivors' Web site, as well as in another variation on a "suddenly single" Web site, and decided to adapt them for our purposes here:

- Denial—This can't be happening; women don't lose their hair.
- Anger—Why is this happening to me when other women have thick, beautiful hair? It's not fair!
- Bargaining—Give me back my hair, and I'll (fill in the blank).
- Depression—I'm really losing my hair. This is hopeless. I'll never find a life partner, be loved, etc., without hair. I can't go on.
- Acceptance—I am more than my hair.

"Own it; live it, shame-free," says Deborah Magids, Ph.D., a psychologist in private practice in New York City. "And then help others to do the same. This can really make a big difference for people."

I had phoned Magids to get some "tips" for dealing with hair loss from a psychologist's point of view, thinking I could create a bulleted, psychological "to do" list for this chapter. But like any good therapist, she helped me see that a set of tips, such as "focus on your strong points," "make a list of positive affirmations," and the like, were little more than lip service if we do not own our hair loss and, through this ownership, find a way to rise above it.

Finding a New Normal

Magids said when dealing with a loss of a part of us, we need to define a new normal. To illustrate this, she shared the fact that she had to do this when diagnosed with celiac disease—the inability to digest gluten, the protein found in wheat and some other grains. "I went into a depression and went through stages of mourning and grief," she told me. "I was never going to eat pizza again. I was never going to eat an Oreo cookie again, or my steamed dumplings or whole-wheat bread. In the scheme of things, giving up gluten and wheat is not a big deal, but it was a complete change of lifestyle and loss of things that I loved. I went through a mourning process."

She says that as a psychologist, understanding this process didn't necessarily make it any simpler. Anything that you have to give up, no matter how small, is a "mini-death," she explains. "Now, given the significance of a woman's hair to her, it's a huge death."

Magids says women losing their hair "need the validation that they're supposed to feel really bad about it. It sucks. And there's not a woman alive who, with the threat of the loss of her hair, wouldn't feel horrible. The worst thing you can say to someone is, 'Oh, please, just get over it and get a wig.'" And the second-worst thing is to offer false hope or fake cures.

Rhani has come to terms with dealing with the loss of her hair. She offers this advice: "You have to realize two things—one, it really is akin to any kind of loss, and two, you won't have the support structure you feel you should. It's how people deal with women's hair loss. They're either going to tell you that you look fine, that you're crazy, or tell you it's just a phase. It's all for good intentions, but you're just not going to get the support for something that's causing you so much actual grief."

Rhani acknowledges the tremendous mental suffering women with hair loss cope with. "You feel like an alien in your life, she says. "I think it's like any challenge or loss. You can come out of it so much richer at the other end, but if you don't realize you're going to have to go through this process, you're going to go through it alone."

Living a Full Life

Just as some people who are, by society's standards, overweight and have embraced the concept of being big and beautiful, we who are suffering from thinning hair or frank baldness can help others deal with it if we can begin to own it ourselves.

Many of the women who wrote to me have embraced their hair loss—not because they have given up, but because after having tried to correct all they can correct, they have gone through the mourning process and have let it go. Even though they may still be searching for that elusive cure, their hair loss has ceased to define their lives.

Laura, twenty, turned her hair loss into a way of helping others like her. After contacting several renowned hair loss experts, she felt empowered to go public. "I created and run HerAlopecia.com, the first and only Web site dedicated solely to women's hair-loss information and support."

"I hate living like this. I hate my wig, I hate my life, and yet, I have learned so much positive about myself through this," says Tracy, thirty-three, who suffers from a rare condition called lichen planopilaris, which causes a patchy hair loss similar to AA. "I have learned how open I can be about myself, and I am very willing to talk with anyone about my hair loss if they ask. By hiding women's hair loss, it creates more of a stigma and makes us all so alone." She adds, "What can we do as a society to help women see that they are not alone? We need support. There is a lot of support for a woman going through cancer, but so little for every other woman."

Caroline, twenty-two, like Tracy, has taken ownership of her hair loss. "I just want to say that losing my hair is a blessing in disguise. It has made me realize all that I do have in life," she told me. "I'm healthy, my loved ones are healthy. It really is just hair, and there are worse things that could affect my appearance, like scars and disabilities." Caroline, however, did not come to her acceptance instantly. She says that as a teenager she harbored thoughts of suicide: "Teenagers aren't supposed to lose their hair. Added to body image and many other pressures and insecurities that normal high school girls have, I was a total mess. I truly believed I was worthless and that no boy would ever find me attractive."

But now she sees even this in a different light. "I call my hair loss 'jerk repellent' because it keeps all the shallow men away from me, and I was able to find a deep, caring, loving boyfriend that loved me for who I am."

Melanie also took steps at a very young age to find ways to cope with her ectodermal dysplasia, a genetic condition that causes hair loss, among other things. During her first year of college, she had to cope with rumors that she had cancer. She said it was difficult to make friends because "all people seemed to see in me was my hair. It was the worst feeling of my life—feeling alone in the world, like no one understood, no one cared, and that everyone viewed me as different. I went to my dorm room and felt as if the world was crashing down on me."

Then Melanie found information on the American Academy of Dermatology Web site about a place called Camp Discovery, for children and teens with skin conditions. Melanie decided to become a volunteer, since alopecia is considered a skin condition. "This was one of the first major steps for rebuilding my self-esteem," Melanie writes in an essay about her condition. She says she really felt like herself for the first time at Camp Discovery. "Now, every summer since 2000, I have been going back to camp, spending two weeks away with my friends where I can truly be me," she says.

Chrissa, thirty-three, who suffers with alopecia areata, found a way to be proactive about her disease by running a golf tournament. "The purpose of our tournament is to promote awareness and support research to help find a cure for alopecia areata through the National Alopecia Areata Foundation and the Boston-area support group," she says. Information about the Links for Locks golf tournament is posted on the NAAF Web site (www.naaf.org).

Getting Rid of the "If Onlys"

These women—and many more like them—are taking bold steps in owning their hair loss and moving on with their lives. It's not easy, and some of us may never be able to be so bold.

I think the biggest obstacle with hair loss is that it keeps so many of us from putting our best foot forward. Hair loss—like being overweight or having serious skin problems —keeps some of us from fulfilling our potential.

We sabotage ourselves with the "if onlys": If only I had thick, luxurious hair, I'd be loved; if only my hair weren't thinning, I could apply for that job; if only I didn't have to wear a wig, I could be a dancer. "The reality," Magids explains, "is that it becomes an excuse. Too many 'if only' sentences, and you're miserable. If you're not paying attention to what you have and being grateful but are just paying attention to what you don't have, you're a very unhappy person. The happier people are just paying more attention to what they have than what they don't have."

Katie, nineteen, has put her hair loss in a positive light. She sought out a renowned hair loss expert and will be doing some research with her as well as seeking help for her own hair loss. But she also decided to do something else.

"The one good thing about my hair loss is that it renewed my desire to be a doctor, because I got so frustrated with the majority of the ones that I saw this summer," she told me. "I felt it was my duty to actually get out there, learn about hair, and be able to treat people."

Sue, thirty-seven, sums up her feelings this way: "My main struggle is the way our society is obsessed by the way people look, and if you look different, then you are almost separated from society. I feel very strongly about women like myself trying to gain the courage to go out there and be ourselves. Men are completely accepted socially when they are bald, but a woman? Sometimes I think people think I am trying to make a statement by being out in public without anything on my head, but this grew out of necessity. I have three small children, and I literally just got to the point where I thought, why can't I just be me?"

She runs a complementary therapy business and teaches Reiki and Indian head massage. "It just seemed like a good joke at the time," she quips.

Dotty, forty-one, told me she wants more education for the public about what it's like to be a bald woman in today's society. "It's very difficult to feel normal when everyone sees a bald woman as some sort of freak or thinks I have cancer," she wrote to me. In her effort to take control of her hair loss, Dotty says that while she has nice wigs, if she doesn't feel like wearing one, she'll just wear a bandanna, and she adds, "I have decided to tattoo my whole head so that when people stare, I give them something to stare at. I already have two tattoos on my head."

Finding Our Voices

People are like stained-glass windows. They sparkle and shine when the sun is out, but when the darkness sets in, their true beauty is revealed only if there is light from within.
—*Elisabeth Kübler-Ross*

One day, I said to my best friend, James: "I fear I'll be totally bald by the time I'm seventy." Without missing a beat, he simply said, "But you have the eyes for it."

It's easy to say we are more than our hair, but it's very difficult to live it on a day-to-day basis, especially in our appearance-conscious society. Gentle reminders from dear friends and loved ones can certainly help, but we need more—we need to open a dialogue about it.

Discussing hair loss is the only way a viable treatment option or the long-sought cure will be found.

I want our inner lights to shine, not our balding pates. I want the shame in being a woman with hair loss to end.

Perhaps we need a slogan and a ribbon or some other symbol that we can stick on the backs of our cars to raise awareness of women's hair loss. Perhaps our "ribbon" is an empty ponytail scrunchy with the words from the 1960s musical *Hair:* "Give me down-to-there hair."

When Melissa Etheridge appeared on the Grammy Awards show in February 2005, she caused quite a stir. In the throes of her battle with breast cancer, she gave an incredibly stunning performance of Janis Joplin's "Piece of My Heart." What did the press and various Web logs say about her performance?

Take a look:

"The brave rocker, who appeared bald . . ." (Contact Music)

"Bald from chemotherapy treatment for breast cancer yet eschewing a wig, she wailed the tar out of Janis Joplin's 'Piece of My Heart'" (*Edmonton Sun*).

"A defiantly bald Melissa Etheridge, recovering from breast cancer . . ." (*Miami Herald Sun*).

"Music's past was given its due without shortchanging the present, and the incomparable Melissa Etheridge demonstrated that one can be rendered bald from cancer-blasting chemotherapy and still have no trouble summoning the spirit of Janis Joplin" (*Hollywood Reporter*).

The *Oregonian* not only adds to the tribute to the courageous Etheridge by titling its article "Bald and Belting It Out," but includes this important and telling paragraph: "Many women say hair loss is the most traumatic part of having cancer—worse than losing a breast or enduring chemotherapy. Losing hair can feel like the equivalent of losing femininity, beauty, and therefore value. Covering up at all costs, even with an itchy wig in summer, is a way many women choose to protect their self-identities and fend off pity during treatment."

Reread that last sentence, especially if you are not dealing with hair loss. How do women "protect their self-identities and fend off pity" when they are suffering from hair loss that is not caused by cancer treatments or other medical conditions?

I was completely taken aback that the media seemed to find Etheridge heroic more for the fact that she dared to appear onstage bald rather than for the fact that she performed while still recovering from a life-threatening illness. Her baldness is symbolic of her struggle with cancer, and I do not want my words to be misconstrued as belittling Etheridge's fight against breast cancer in any way. Her performance was indeed heroic.

Etheridge spoke about her decision to do the performance sans wig during an interview with Stone Phillips on NBC's *Dateline.* Phillips asked if Etheridge ever considered wearing a wig, and she answered: "Oh, I never considered wearing a wig. I can't imagine putting a wig on. And I couldn't imagine a wig staying on my head as I was flying around that stage."

For those of us dealing with hair loss, Etheridge's performance is bittersweet. We cannot help being struck by the fact that for a woman to appear bald in public is seen as very brave—within the context of fighting a life-threatening disease.

What about women who are simply dealing with baldness that is not temporary? What about the everyday heroes—women who go out in public each day with thinning hair or frank balding patches?

I notice celebrities on talk shows whose hair is carefully coifed to hide thinness, or who are likely wearing extensions or using other camouflage methods, or who are simply out there, with painfully thin hair. While I'd like to mention names, it is not my place to "out" these people. But wouldn't it be terrific if even one celebrity talked about coping with thinning hair or hair loss? If one in four women are dealing with it, it cannot have bypassed Hollywood and Broadway.

Phyllis Diller, the comedienne with the wild hair and kooky outfits who does sidesplitting routines about her husband "Fang," did something amazingly brave in the

1970s. Diller has been very open through the years about her several face-lifts. One day, on a daytime talk show, she gave viewers a behind-the-scenes view of how she transforms herself through wigs and makeup. She began with no makeup and no eyelashes, and her hair, as I recall, is painfully thin. In a word, she looked like anything but herself and not very pretty. She took the viewers through the steps, from her bare face to makeup to eyelashes to wig. It was stunning, and it was brave. By doing this, Diller showed millions of American women how to make the most of what they have. We also got to see the otherwise whacky Diller as an incredible beautiful woman, inside and out.

In the September 2002 issue of *More* magazine, Jamie Lee Curtis took on the Hollywood illusion of perfection and showed us that it is indeed done with smoke, mirrors, and damn good lighting. "There's a reality to the way I look without my clothes on," she said. "I don't have great thighs. I have very big breasts and a soft, fat little tummy. And I've got back fat. People assume that I'm walking around in little spaghetti-strap dresses. It's insidious—Glam Jamie, the Perfect Jamie, the great figure, blah, blah, blah. And I don't want the unsuspecting 40-year-old women of the world to think that I've got it going on. It's such a fraud. And I'm the one perpetuating it."

Well, who knew?

Wouldn't it be great if one of the actresses with less-than-perfect hair, or who is as terrified as we are of going completely bald, went public with it as Jamie Lee did about her figure imperfections? Wouldn't it be great for someone in the public eye to talk of the heartache of trying things to regrow hair with little or no results? Or talk of fearing for her career because of her hair? Or simply bare the dirty little secret of her balding head?

The American Academy of Dermatology has designated August as Hair Loss Awareness Month. We need to help ourselves and others cast off the shame of living with hair loss by airing our true feelings about it.

Maybe just say out loud to the one person you most trust: "I'm losing my hair, and it really scares me."

Resources

For Further Information about Hair Loss

Alopecia Areata Registry
http://www.alopeciaareataregistry.org

American Academy of Dermatology
Phone: 866-503-SKIN (7546)
http://www.aad.org

American Association of Clinical Endocrinologists
http://www.aace.com

The American College of Obstetricians and Gynecologists
http://www.acog.org

American Osteopathic College of Dermatology
Phone: 800-449-2623
http://www.aocd.org/

European Hair research Society
http://www/ehrs.org

National Alopecia Areata Foundation
Phone: 415-472-3780
http://www.naaf.org

North American Hair Research Society
http://www.nahrs.org

Hair Restoration Surgery Information

American Society of Dermatologic Surgery
http://www.asds-net.org/Patients/factsheets/patients
-Fact_Sheet-hair_rest.html

Bosley Medical Center
http://www.bosley.com

The Foundation for Hair Restoration
http://foundhair.com/

International Society for Hair Restoration Surgery
http://www.ishrs.org

Online Places for Support and Information

HairLossTalk.com
(information, support forums, interviews with hair loss
experts)
http://www.hairlosstalk.com

HerAlopecia.com
(the first women-only hair loss Web site; sister site of Hair
ossTalk; help, support forums, information)
http://www.heralopecia.com

Keratin.com
(good and credible source for information and support)
http://www.keratin.com

Women's Institute for Fine and Thinning Hair
(Don't discount this one because it's from Pfizer [maker
of Rogaine]; it's quite informative)
http://www.womenshairinstitute.com

Resources for Dietary Information

American Dietetic Association
http://www.eatright.org

Institute of Medicine of the National Academies
(see the Web site for the Dietary Reference Intake Table)
Phone: 202-334-2352
http://www.iom.edu

National Institutes of Health Office of Dietary
Supplements
http://ods.od.nih.gov

U.S. Food and Drug Administration
http://www.fda.gov

Complementary and Alternative Medicines (CAM)

Alternative Medicine Foundation
http://www.amfoundation.org

HerbMed (database on herbal medicines)
http://www.herbmed.org

Memorial Sloan-Kettering Cancer Center's Integrative
Medicine Service
(for information on herbs, botanicals, and other products)
http://www.mskcc.org/mskcc/html/11571.cfm?
recordid=426

University of Washington School of Medicine, Department
of Family Medicine
www.fammed.washington.edu/predoctoral/CAM/sites
.html

Research and Information on Hair Loss and Related Health Conditions

eMedicine
(good database for basic information)
http://www.emedicine.com/derm

Entrez PubMed
(for finding abstracts of clinical trials)
http://www.ncbi.nlm.nih.gov/entrez/query.fcgi?

MerckSource Health Information
http://www.mercksource.com/pp/us/cns/cns_home.jsp

The National Institutes of Health's Medline Plus
Encyclopedia
http://www.nlm.nih.gov/medlineplus/encyclopedia.html

Some Other Web Sites Worth Checking Out

Camp Discovery
(a camp for children with alopecia areata or other hair
loss and skin diseases)
http://www.campdiscovery.org/Camp_Discovery.htm

Links for Locks
(information on the golf tournament to raise research
money)
http://www.naaf.org/LinksForLocks/linksforlocks.asp

Resources for Hats, Scarves, Wigs, and Cover-Up Products

American Hair Loss Council
(good place to start if you're considering hair additions,
extensions, or wigs; provides a good overview on hair loss
in general, plus a listing of salons that adhere to their
code of conduct)
http://www.ahlc.org

Just In Time
(A great resource for those days you just don't want to
cope with it. While touted for women with AA or hair loss
from chemotherapy, these hats are lovely for anyone.)
http://www.softhats.com

National Areata Alopecia Marketplace
http://www.naaf.org/marketplace/marketplace.asp

 *B*

Alternative Medicine

With alternative medicines, the risks as well as the benefits in using them may not be well known, if known at all. And often the Web sites and other places touting their benefits will bolster their argument by saying these ingredients have been used in folk medicine for hundreds of years. The sites are often more weighted toward what the nutrients can do than what they cannot do or their possible side effects.

Remember vitamins, herbs, and other supplements, just like pharmaceuticals, are big business. Nearly every time you do a Google search on any aspect of hair loss, there are hundreds of sites willing to give you information and sell you "treatments."

How can you determine if the vitamins, minerals, herbs, and other supplements are safe and, moreover, effective? It's not easy.

The Dietary Supplement Health and Education Act of 1994 (DSHEA) allows dietary supplements to be sold without the premarket safety evaluations required of other new food ingredients, and says they may carry "structure/function" claims.

Under DSHEA, dietary supplements may make statements of nutritional support if the company can substantiate the statement as truthful and not misleading, and if they notify the FDA within thirty days after first marketing the supplement. The label on such supplements must prominently display: "This statement has not been evaluated by the Food and Drug Administration. This product is not intended to diagnose, treat, cure or prevent any disease."

Some examples of structure/function claims are "helps maintain cholesterol levels," "helps support cartilage and joint function," and "improves absentmindedness." Those not permissible under DSHEA as a structure/function claim include "lowers cholesterol," "inhibits platelet aggregation," and "maintains bone density in postmenopausal women."

But we do see such claims, don't we? This is because there is a law that allows some foods and supplements to use such wording, the American Dietetic Association (ADA) says. According to the ADA, the Nutrition Labeling and Education Act (NLEA) of 1990 allows health claims that "describe a relationship between a food substance and a disease or other related condition (i.e., a 'risk reduction' relationship)," and only if "significant scientific agreement among qualified experts exists about the validity of the relationship described in that claim." Only thirteen such health claims are currently approved by the FDA. One example is calcium products with the FDA-approved wording, "Regular exercise and a healthful diet with enough calcium help teens and young adult white and Asian American women maintain good bone health and may reduce their risk of osteoporosis." Such health claims carry a great body of evidence behind them.

The ADA notes that foods carrying "an FDA-approved health claim (sterol/stanol esters, oats, psyllium, soy) generally are supported by two dozen or more well-designed published clinical trials."

The yet-to-be finalized and passed FDA Modernization Act of 1997 will allow expedited health claims if they are based on current, published authoritative statements from predefined scientific bodies, such as the touting of whole grains in the prevention of heart disease and cancer, and in December 2002 the agency said "qualified health claims" will be allowed such as this one: "Selenium and cancer: Selenium may reduce the risk of certain cancers. . . . FDA has determined that this evidence is limited and not conclusive."

If you are a person at risk for or suffering from cancer, which part of this labeling do you see? The part that says it's inconclusive or the part that says "may reduce the risk"? Remember this when looking at such claims or even less qualified claims on so-called hair remedies or supplements touted for hair loss.

Online Purchasing

Herbs and supplements that you can purchase online should trigger an alarm bell. Their labels may be within the legal limits of what they can say, but read between the lines.

Consider this statistic offered by the American Cancer Society: In 2003, U.S. poison control centers had almost sixty-two thousand calls related to supplements such as vitamins or herbs, with over one thousand severe outcomes and seven deaths.

Before taking supplements check them out on reputable Web sites such as:

- Memorial Sloan-Kettering's Integrative Medicine Service (www.mskcc.org)

- The National Center for Complementary and Alternative Medicine (http://nccam.nih.gov)
- The Medline Plus Medical Encyclopedia (http://www.nlm.nih.gov/medlineplus/encyclopedia.html)
- United States Pharmacopeia (http://www.uspdqi.org)
- Hair Loss Talk and Her Alopecia (http://www.hairlosstalk.com and http://www.her alopecia.com), which both regularly update readers about the latest alternative treatments for hair loss, including nutrients, and are a good resource.

The USP Label

In 1997 the U.S. Pharmacopeia (USP) began publishing guidelines or standards of strength, quality, purity, packaging, and labeling to assure a uniform quality control for supplements. Manufacturers voluntarily agree to adhere to these standards by affixing the USP label on their packaging.

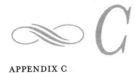

Topical Minoxidil

At some point in dealing with your hair loss, you will undoubtedly try topical minoxidil. It is sold commercially, without a prescription, as Rogaine, and it is also available in less expensive generic versions.

This potassium-channel opener and vasodilator began its life as a treatment for high blood pressure. In 1988, 2 percent topical minoxidil solution, sold under the name Rogaine, was approved for use as a treatment for men with male pattern hair loss. In 1996, it was approved for use without a prescription by both men and women for the treatment of genetic or pattern hair loss. A 5 percent solution was approved, in 1997, for use in men, and while not approved as a treatment for women, because it is available without a prescription, some women use it and have found it more beneficial for their hair loss than the lower dosage.

Advertisements for Rogaine, featuring models with tresses most of us with hair loss can only dream about, make it seem as if the product will work for everyone in restoring a full head of hair.

For many people, it will not work at all.

However, before you discount this treatment, although hair regrowth occurs in only a small percentage of women using minoxidil, it does appear to at least maintain the hair they have and thicken the hair shaft a bit for most people. Nearly every doctor I interviewed said that topical minoxidil is a mainstay of treatment. They also said that the earlier you begin using it, the better.

Is it a cure? No.

Is it a stopgap measure? Possibly.

Frequently Asked Questions about Topical Minoxidil

Q. Is topical minoxidil safe?

A. It is probably one of the safer treatments for hair loss. The main side effect with its use is hypertrichosis, or excessive hair growth, usually on the face. This affects 3 to 5 percent of women using the 2 percent solution, and more than 5 percent of those using the 5 percent dosage. Hypertrichosis will usually disappear after a year even if you continue to use minoxidil. If you stop the treatment, it will abate within one to six months.

Q. My scalp itches, and it seems as if I am having more hair shedding than before I began treatment with minoxidil.

A. Hair shedding at the beginning of treatment happens in some people. Sometimes the telogen phase of hair growth is accelerated. While disconcerting, this is usually temporary.

Scalp itching can be due to the propylene glycol base that minoxidil is suspended in, and a dermatologist or a compounding pharmacist can put the active ingredient of the treatment in a less-irritating base, such as polyethylene glycol. Some dermatologists prescribe a topical steroid to help control the itch. However, since this will likely add to its expense, you could try calming the itch with either ketoconazole (Nizoral shampoo) or Tricomin shampoo or spray; both of these treatments may also help with hair loss.

Q. When should I see results?
A. You should see some results with topical minoxidil within four months of use. For this or any treatment, experts say you must give it at least this amount of time to see if it will have any effect, and some even suggest you need a full year to assess its efficacy.

Q. Should I use 2 percent or 5 percent?
A. If you are seeing good results with 2 percent minoxidil, there probably isn't any reason to try 5 percent. If you have not seen any results with 2 percent, the higher dosage may help, so before deciding the treatment doesn't work at all, give it a try. However, the chance of side effects is greater with the higher dosage.

Q. Can I use minoxidil if I am pregnant or plan to get pregnant?
A. If you are using minoxidil or contemplating using it and are planning to get pregnant or are pregnant, talk with your obstetrician or gynecologist about the risks of using it while pregnant.

Q. What does minoxidil cost?
A. It used to be that Pfizer's Rogaine was the only commercially available version of topical minoxidil, but now there are also generic brands, and this has helped lower the cost of the treatment. Typically, the cost of topical minoxidil is between $10 and $20 for a one-month supply. You can also find it bundled in three-month packages at a discounted quantity price.
  NOTE: There have been anecdotal reports that the generic versions of minoxidil are not as effective as the

branded version. I suggest trying both and seeing which one works best for you. If money is a consideration, you might try the generic first. If you don't see results in a few months, try the branded product (Rogaine) before quitting topical minoxidil completely.

Q. How is minoxidil applied?
A. Minoxidil must be applied to the scalp twice a day, morning and evening. One dropperful is applied directly to the scalp and massaged in.

Q. Is minoxidil a life sentence?
A. The harsh reality of topical minoxidil is that if you stop using it, your hair will return to its previous state—you're right back where you started. This is the most discouraging aspect of the treatment and one to which many women are unwilling to commit.

Tips for Using Topical Minoxidil

- Apply directly to thinning or bald areas of the scalp, rub in, and let dry.
- Do not comb your hair before it dries, or you will draw it through your hair and make your hair greasy. After the scalp dries, it is fine to style your hair as usual and use styling products such as volumizing gels, mousses, sprays, etc. If these work best on wet hair, rewet your hair.
- Apply minoxidil an hour or so before bedtime to lessen the chance of it getting on your pillow, which can increase the chance of facial hypertrichosis.
- If you wear contact lenses, put them in before you apply the minoxidil. (Trust me on this one!)
- Take a "before" picture of the thinning areas of your scalp; then take photos at four months, six

months, and a year to objectively document your progress.

- If you have an important event and you just don't like the way your hair looks when you use the treatment, skip the morning's treatment and style your hair optimally, then get back to the regimen that night and the following days. I do this and haven't seen any adverse results. However, do not go more than a day or so without the treatment.

- Calm itching or irritation with Tricomin or Nizoral shampoo or Tricomin spray. Or ask your physician or compounding pharmacist about reformulating minoxidil in a less-irritating base.

- Do not use topical minoxidil on the days when you color or perm your hair.

- Be sure to ask your physician: "What other treatment options might we try if Rogaine doesn't work for me?"

Bibliography

Chapter 3

Bhorjee, Anita. "10 Hair Loss Myths." Unpublished manuscript, used with permission.

Boss, Angela, S.E. Weidman, and R.S. Legro. *Living With PCOS.* Omaha, Neb.: Addicus Books, 2001.

Cheung, Theresa. *Androgen Disorders in Women: The Most Neglected Hormone Problem.* Alameda, Calif.: Hunter House, 1999.

Cuellar, M. L., O. Gluck, J. F. Molina, S. Gutierrez, C. Garcia, and R. Espinoza. "Silicone Breast Implant-Associated Musculoskeletal Manifestations." *Journal of Clinical Rheumatology* 14, no. 6 (1995): 667–72.

Dobke, M. K., J. K. Svahn, V. L. Vastine, B. N. Landon, P. C. Stein, and C. L. Parsons. "Characterization of Microbial Presence at the Surface of Silicone Mammary Implants." Annals of Plastic Surgery 34, no. 6 (June 1995): 563–71.

Hannapel, Coriene. "Facelift Aftershock Alleviated." *Dermatology Times,* June 1, 2002.

Hordinsky, Maria. "Hair Loss." *Best Practice of Medicine,* June 2003.

Jesitus, John. "Identify Underlying Condition to Treat Women's Hair Loss." *Cosmetic Surgery Times.* Oct 1, 2001.

Minkin, J., and T. Hanlon. "Talk to the Doctor." *Prevention* 54, no. 3 (March 2002): 156.

National Alopecia Areata Foundation. "Frequently Asked Questions." http://www.naaf.org/requestinfo/faq.asp.

Ostermeyer Shoaib, B., and B. M. Patten. "Human Adjuvant Disease: Presentation as a Multiple Sclerosis-like Syndrome." *Southern Medicine Journal* 89, no. 2 (February 1996): 179–88.

Sawaya, M. E., and J. Shapiro. "Alopecia: Unapproved Treatments or Indications." *American Journal of Clinical Dermatology,* March–April 2000: 177–86.

Shapiro, Jerry. *Hair Loss: Principles of Diagnosis and Management of Alopecia.* London: Martin Dunitz, 2002.

Westman, E. C., et al. "Effect of 6-Month Adherence to a Very Low Carbohydrate Diet Program." *American Journal of Medicine* 113 (2002): 30–36.

Chapter 4

Hunt, N., and S. McHale. "The Psychological Impact of Alopecia." *British Medical Journal* 331 (October 22, 2005): 951–53.

Van Der Donk, J., J. S. Hunfeld, J. Passchier, K. J.Knegt-Junk, and C. Nieboer. "Quality of Life and Maladjustment Associated with Hair Loss in Women with Alopecia Androgenetica." *Social Science Medicine* 38 (January 1994): 159–63

Williamson, D., M. Gonzalez, A. Y. Finlay. "The Effect of Hair Loss on quality of Life." *Journal of the European Academy of Dermatology and Venereology* 15 March 2000: 137–9.

Chapter 5

Springer, K., M. Brown, and D. L. Stulberg. "Common Hair Disorders." *American Family Physician* 68 (July 1, 2003): 93–102.

Chapter 6

American Society of Health-System Pharmacists. "MedlinePlus Drug Information: Flutamide." http://www.nlm.nih.gov/medlineplus/druginfo/medmaster/a697045.html.

Bandaranayake, L., and P. Mirmirani. "Hair Loss Remedies: Separating Fact from Fiction." *Cutis* 73, no. 2 (February 2004): 107–14.

Bhorjee, Anita. "10 Hair Loss Myths." Unpublished manuscript, used with permission.

Callender, V. D., A. J. McMichael, and G. F. Cohen. "Medical and Surgical Therapies for Alopecias in Black Women." *Dermatologic Therapy* 17 (2004): 164–76.

Haber, R. S. "Pharmacologic Management of Pattern Hair Loss." *Facial Plastic Surgery Clinics of North America* 12, no. 2 (May 2004): 181–89.

Happle, R., K. Cebulla, K. Echternacht-Happle "Dinitrochlorobenzene Therapy for Alopecia Areata." *Archives of Dermatology* 114, no. 11 (November 1978).

Mayo Clinic. "Hair Loss: Cancer-Related Causes and How to Cope." Reprinted by St. Anthony's Medical Center. January 2004. http://www.stanthonysmedcenter.com/mayo/parsexmldisplay.asp?xd=CA00037.

National Alopecia Areata Foundation. "Medical Questions and Answers." http://www.naaf.org/research/research-q_and_a-treatments.asp.

Pierard-Franchimont, C., P. De Doncker, G. Cauwenbergh, and G. E. Pierard. "Ketoconazole Shampoo:

Effect of Long-Term Use in Androgenic Alopecia." *Dermatology* 196, no. 4 (1998): 474–77.

Sawaya, M. E., and J. Shapiro. "Alopecia: Unapproved Treatments or Indications." *American Journal of Clinical Dermatology,* March–April 2000: 177–86.

Shapiro, Jerry. "Treatment of Alopecia Areata (AA) with Special Emphasis on Topical Immunotherapy with Diphenylcyclopropenone (DCP)." *Skin Therapy Letter,* August 1996.

Springer, K., M. Brown, and D. L. Stulberg. "Common Hair Disorders." *American Family Physician* 68 (July 1, 2003).

Thiedke, Carolyn C. "Alopecia in Women." *American Family Physician* 67, no. 5 (March 1, 2003): 1007–14.

Women's Health Initiative. "Questions and Answers about the WHI Postmenopausal Hormone Therapy Trials." April 2004. http://www.nhlbi.nih.gov/whi/whi_faq.htm.

Chapter 7

Callender, V. D., A. J. McMichael, and G. F. Cohen. "Medical and Surgical Therapies for Alopecias in Black Women." *Dermatologic Therapy* 17 (2004).

Chapter 8

Roberts, Janet. "Ironing Out One of the Many Causes of Hair Loss in Women." *Environmental Nutrition* 27, no.7 (July 2004): 7.

Kantor, J., L. J. Kessler, D. G. Brooks, and G. Cotsarelis. "Decreased Serum Ferritin Is Associated with Alopecia in Women." *Journal of Investigative Dermatology* 121, no. 5 (November 2003): 985–88.

Roberts, Janet L. "Examining the Etiology of Telogen Effluvium in Pre- and Postmenopausal Women: A

Chart Review Study." Presented to Third Intercontinental Meeting of Hair Research Societies. June 13–15, 2001. http://www.ehrs.org/conferenceabstracts/2001 tokyo/researchabstracts/157-roberts.htm.

Shapiro, Jerry. *Hair Loss: Principles of Diagnosis and Management of Alopecia.* London: Martin Dunitz, 2002.

Sinclair, R. "There Is No Clear Association between Low Serum Ferritin and Chronic Diffuse Telogen Hair Loss." *British Journal of Dermatology* 147 (2002): 982–84.

Chapter 9

Bandaranayake, L., and P. Mirmirani. "Hair Loss Remedies: Separating Fact from Fiction." *Cutis* 73, no. 2 (February 2004).

Natural Standard and Harvard Medical School Faculty. "Evening Primrose Oil (Oenothera biennis)." Aetna InteliHealth. June 2005. http://www.intelihealth.com/IH/ihtIH/WSIHW000/8513/31402/346441.html?d=dmtContent.

Sawaya, M. E., and J. Shapiro. "Alopecia: Unapproved Treatments or Indications." *American Journal of Clinical Dermatology,* March–April 2000: 177–86.

Chapter 10

Bhorjee, Anita. "10 Hair Loss Myths." Unpublished manuscript, used by permission.

"HairMax LaserComb Cleared for Prevention of Hair Loss and Stimulation of Hair Regrowth in Men and Women by Health Canada." *Business Wire,* January 15, 2003.

Satino, John L., and Michael Markou. "Hair Regrowth and Increased Hair Tensile Strength Using the Hair-Max LaserComb for Low-Level Laser Therapy." *Inter-*

national Journal of Cosmetic Surgery and Aesthetic Dermatology 5, no. 2 (August 2003): 113–17.

Chapter 11

Claudinot, S., M. Nicolas, H. Oshima, A. Rochat, Y. Barrandon. "Long-Term Renewal of Hair Follicles from Clonogenic Multipotent Stem Cells." Proceedings of the National Academy of Sciences of the U.S.A. 102, no. 41 (October 11, 2005): 14677–82.
Cooley, J. "Follicular Cell Implantation: An Update on 'Hair Follicle Cloning.'" *Facial Plastic Surgery Clinics of North America* 12, no. 2 (May 2004): 219–24.

Appendix C

Haber, R. S. "Pharmacologic Management of Pattern Hair Loss." *Facial Plastic Surgery Clinics of North America* 12, no. 2 (May 2004): 181–89.
Thiedke, Carolyn C. "Alopecia in Women." *American Family Physician* 67, no. 5 (March 1, 2003): 1007–14.

Index